+3

J.O.

# A Practical Guide to
# Cataract and Lens Implant Surgery

# A Practical Guide to Cataract and Lens Implant Surgery

## R. S. Bartholomew

BA, MB, BChir(Cantab), FRCS(Edin)

Senior Lecturer, Department of Ophthalmology,
University of Edinburgh; Honorary Consultant
Ophthalmologist, Royal Infirmary, Edinburgh

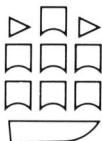

CHURCHILL LIVINGSTONE
EDINBURGH LONDON MELBOURNE AND NEW YORK 1986

CHURCHILL LIVINGSTONE
Medical Division of Longman Group UK Limited

Distributed in the United States of America by Churchill
Livingstone Inc., 1560 Broadway, New York, N.Y. 10036, and
by associated companies, branches and representatives
throughout the world.

First published 1986

ISBN 0 443 03637 3

British Library Cataloguing in Publication Data

Library of Congress Cataloging in Publication Data

Produced by Longman Singapore Publishers (Pte) Ltd.
Printed in Singapore

# Contents

TO ELISABETH

# Foreword

Even when intracapsular cataract extraction had become well established in the 1950s, some older surgeons would say they hoped that, if they ever had cataracts, an extracapsular extraction could be done: there is great comfort in an intact posterior capsule. That verdict is strongly supported by the modern method very ably used by R. Shayle Bartholomew and described in this volume. Consistent success is essential before insertion of intraocular lenses.

The now senior surgeons should not find much difficulty in transferring their affections to the new extracapsular techniques, provided they pay attention to the many details recorded here and so clearly illustrated by the author himself. They will already have the advantage of long practice with the operation microscope and fine instruments, needles and sutures. Capsulotomy by the neodymium YAG laser is another strong incentive for the reluctant changeling who has anxiety about the risks of surgical incision of residual capsule with a knife needle.

This inexpensive volume will be of great value and interest to everyone involved with cataract surgery.

Calbert I. Phillips

# Acknowledgements

I would like to thank all those friends, colleagues and students who by their questions and discussion stimulated me to write this book. I owe a debt of gratitude to John Robertson for his patience and advice on preparation of the manuscript and to Ian Lennox for his encouragement and advice with my illustrations. I must also thank Katharine Watts, Publisher, for her enthusiasm to publish my work.

# 1

# Introduction

The idea of producing a practical guide to extracapsular extraction developed during a number of courses I have run on the subject. Comments from many colleagues and residents suggest that there is a genuine need for such a guide.

Residents have the advantage of being exposed over a number of years to these techniques. They participate closely in the preoperative selection and preparation of the patients. They watch and assist surgeons who are skilled in the techniques and have the valuable experience of seeing and managing operative and postoperative complications. The resident also makes his first practical steps into extracapsular surgery under close supervision. Ideal conditions can be guaranteed for his first attempts and each part of the procedure can be practised in isolation. Should difficulties occur then the experienced surgeon is there to complete the operation successfully for the patient and to relieve the resident from unnecessary psychological trauma.

The surgeon, already experienced in the techniques of the intracapsular method, is increasingly under pressure to embark upon extracapsular surgery. He has none of the advantages of the resident. He has to start by abandoning his hard won technique, one in which he excels, to learn a completely new technique. He must then put it into full effect immediately, taking full responsibility for his patients and for any complications that may ensue. This is indeed a challenge.

How is he to gain the necessary preliminary experience? He can read books — and there are many excellent ones. He may attend courses on extracapsular surgery and lens implantation or he may visit other surgeons at work. He will obviously gain useful knowledge and information

but is likely to come away with many of his questions unanswered and he may not have ready access to anyone able to help him.

This practical guide is an attempt to answer the questions and problems that I myself have had in learning the techniques, and many of the learners' difficulties that have arisen during my teaching courses.

The increase in the popularity of the extracapsular method has been brought about through developments in intraocular lens implantation, particularly by the understanding of operative and postoperative complications.

An intact posterior capsule protects the eye from future retinal detachment and cystoid macular oedema. It reduces irido- and phakodonesis by increasing implant stability. It offers the option of implanting a lens wholly into the posterior chamber. This position — especially if a single plane lens is used — reduces operative trauma to both the cornea and iris. A posterior chamber lens also gives freedom to the pupil to dilate or constrict fully. Examination and treatment of retinal conditions are therefore possible. The implant, close to the nodal point of the eye, is placed at the optimal optical position. An intact posterior capsule offers resistance to the spread of infection.

It is not surprising that a procedure with so many advantages has a number of drawbacks. The extracapsular method is undoubtedly more difficult. It is a longer procedure and involves more manipulation. This causes more trauma to the cornea and iris than occurs with the intracapsular technique. Corneal decompensation and iritis are therefore more frequent. Residual lens material, and there is always some residual lens material, which is normally sequestrated from the body's immunological system, acts as an irritant and allergen and further promotes uveitis. The capsule, clear after operation, becomes opaque in a significant number of patients. A second operation then becomes necessary.

In addition to these normal problems of extracapsular surgery there are the inevitable complications during surgery — tearing of the posterior capsule and rupture of the vitreous face with consequent vitreous loss.

There are no particularly difficult physical manoeuvres to master. The secret is to string together a sequence of operative procedures — none inherently difficult on its own — to produce a satisfactory result. It requires an infinite capacity for taking pains. Each step in the procedure has a marked effect on those that follow. An accumulation of small errors can rapidly lead to an impossible situation where the operation cannot be brought to a satisfactory conclusion.

The surgeon attempting to master the extracapsular technique must be an accomplished user of the operation microscope. Ideally the microscope should have coaxial illumination and should incorporate a variable zoom magnification, fine focus adjustment and a movable field — X/Y shift. The field of view should be as wide as possible. All the controls must be foot operated. Use of the microscope should become an unconscious activity. The correct magnification, focus and field should instantly be chosen for the particular task in hand. The surgeon's hands and mind will thus be freed to concentrate on the problem before him. The extracapsular technique will take longer than the intracapsular even when performed smoothly. One must try therefore not to lengthen it any further by having to fiddle around with the microscope. This not only wastes valuable time but is likely further to obscure one's view through the cornea — corneal haze — and allow the pupil to constrict further. This jeopardizes one's chances of clear observation.

Clear observation at all stages is the second and most important requirement for the extracapsular surgeon. He must be able to see the various ocular structures before he can identify them. Instant recognition of these various structures — anterior capsule, cortical fibres, posterior capsule, vitreous face, capsular flaps and tears — is essential before a satisfactory operation can be done with any confidence.

# 2

# Indications

The general indication for extracapsular cataract extraction has been that of age. In younger people, where the hyaloid capsular attachment is strong, some form of extracapsular removal has usually been carried out. The old practices of needling, linear extraction or simple extracapsular removal without use of the microscope bear little resemblance to today's aspiration, irrigation/aspiration or phakoemulsification carried out under direct microscopic control.

The indications now are closely bound up with the indications for lens implantation. The surgeon contemplating extracapsular surgery will probably already be implanting lenses of various types following on from intracapsular extractions. His patients will mainly be elderly. He will therefore be considering an extracapsular extraction on most of his patients. This may seem to be an exaggeration. However, the scope and range of lens implantation have rapidly increased and will continue to do so. The surgeon like myself, who a few years ago only considered an implant in a patient over seventy years of age, now considers every adult patient. There are of course some surgeons who also implant lenses into children. The important point to make is that the results of extracapsular extractions are so good that they can now be offered to most patients. Surgeons will therefore find themselves doing extracapsular extractions in the future when, at the moment, intracapsular extractions are very much the norm.

My indications are now similar to those for lens implantation, when I consider every patient. Absolute contraindications to an implant include growing children, uveitis — past or active and heterochromic cyclitis — and uncontrolled glaucoma. Relative contraindications include controlled glaucoma, corneal endothelial disease, an only eye, a failed implant in the other eye, cystoid macula oedema in the other eye, high myopia, diabetes and retinal detachment.

The indications for extracapsular extraction without implant include high myopia, previous retinal detachment in either eye, uveitis or heterochromic cyclitis in younger patients and children. I expect that my indications for extracapsular extraction and lens implantation will widen over the next few years.

## Children

There are good reasons for considering a lens implant in children who have had a traumatic cataract in one eye, or where congenital cataract threatens to cause amblyopia and permanent visual loss. One might say, 'What is there to lose?'. These patients are perhaps best treated in a centre able to specialize in this restricted field. I should prefer the less experienced implant surgeon not to attempt these cases.

## Uveitis

Uveitis is one of the main complications of the extracapsular method. A persistent or recurrent uveitis may lead to permanent deposits on the surface of the implant, posterior synechiae, thickening and opacity of the posterior capsule, glaucoma and possible damage to the corneal endothelium and macula. It is therefore sensible not to contemplate a lens implant in such patients. An extracapsular extraction may of course be indicated in the younger patient with uveitis and cataract without an implant.

## Glaucoma

Uncontrolled glaucoma is an obvious contraindication. The glaucoma must be controlled first. If it is readily controlled medically, subsequent extracapsular extraction and lens implantation can be done. Control using pilocarpine will complicate the extraction, however, and postoperative use of steroids may cause temporary difficulties with a pronounced hypertensive response. The beginner is advised not to attempt such cases.

## Corneal endothelial disease

The patient with obvious Fuch's dystrophy, marked cornea guttata or where the corneal endothelium has probably been damaged — trauma, previous operations, open angle glaucoma with or without drainage operation, angle closure glaucoma where there has been an acute congestive attack or an iridectomy has been done — should all be treated with caution. It is better to leave these higher risk eyes until one's extracapsular technique has been perfected. If corneal cell counts can be done then a cut-off point of 1000 cells/sq.mm is advised.

## An only eye

The surgeon should give the patient the technique in which he is most confident. It is far better to have a good intracapsular extraction than a botched-up extracapsular one, with or without an implant.

## A failed implant in the other eye

The reasons for the failure will have to be examined before deciding on the procedure best suited for the second or 'only' eye. The deciding factor should again be the confidence of the surgeon in his own method.

## Cystoid macular oedema

The occurrence of cystoid macular oedema in the first eye is a positive indication for an extracapsular extraction in the second eye. Care should be exercised when cystoid macular oedema is more likely to occur — as in diabetic and other retinopathies.

## High myopia and previous retinal detachment

High myopia or a previous retinal detachment in either eye are both indications for an extracapsular extraction. The risk of subsequent retinal detachment is thereby reduced. It is especially important in these patients to be able to observe the fundus after the operation. The pupil must dilate and the central and peripheral capsule remain clear. An implant may be an additional bar to clear observation of the retina and may therefore be contraindicated.

## Diabetes

Proliferative retinopathy and rubeosis iridis are contraindications to a lens implant. Diabetes, usually the adult onset type, without such changes, is no contraindication. The macular degeneration frequently present in such patients makes them poor candidates for aphakic spectacles, and a lens implant is of considerable optical help, as in senile macular degeneration. The pupil must be free to dilate and the media sufficiently clear to observe the fundus and to deliver any necessary coagulation treatment.

The main thrust of this practical guide will be towards the performance of an extracapsular cataract extraction for senile cataract with the intention of proceding to a posterior chamber lens implant using a single plane modified J-loop type of lens, placed in the eye without a capsular bag. The methods to be described are therefore limited to a didactic presentation of the author's method. It is certainly not the only method and it may well not be the best method. It is, however, a method now widely used and one which produces good results and I therefore have no hesitation in presenting it. I must however stress that this whole field of surgery is undergoing rapid change. I often try out minor modifications in technique. Some of these I abandon; others I incorporate into my preferred method. You should do the same thing: select those features which suit and thereby build up your own system.

# 3

# Assessment

The assessment of the patient will include a general history and examination with the object of deciding whether a local or general anaesthetic is advisable and whether the patient's health requires a period of treatment prior to the operation. Where there is any doubt it is wiser to delay the operation until the patient's health has been improved as much as possible. Many patients with senile cataract have chronic illness — heart disease, respiratory disease, diabetes and other problems are frequently encountered — and it may be necessary to operate when the patient is far from fit. The anaesthetist will certainly inform you as to whether the individual is fit for a general. You must however be prepared to undertake the procedure under a local if necessary. You must remember that the extracapsular procedure will take considerably longer than the intracapsular one and that the fine controlled manipulations may be exceedingly difficult in a restless patient under local anaesthesia. I should advise the beginner to start his extracapsular operations under a good general anaesthetic, and therefore to choose his patient accordingly.

The routine history and examination of the eyes should include all that is necessary from the ocular point of view. There are however a number of aspects of which you should take particular note.

First of all the past ocular history. Beware of the uniocular cataract particularly, in the patient who is in a younger age group. Ask about previous injuries to the eye, often long forgotten, or the possibility of uveitis. Examine carefully for any signs of trauma — minute tears in the pupil margin, alterations in the iris architecture, for example — look for any difference in iris colour and a possible heterochromic cyclitis.

Examine the corneal endothelium by specular reflection for possible changes. It is better to discover any such changes before operation rather than after.

Remember glaucoma. Enquire about a family history. Take note of the ocular pressure and be particularly wary about pressure levels around the upper limit of normal. It may not be possible to assess the optic disc or field of vision in the presence of a cataract. Therefore check the pressure again, ideally early in the morning. An unsuspected glaucoma of the open angle variety may give you postoperative problems with steroid treatment. Pseudocapsular exfoliation is to be noted, with pupil dilated. There is an obvious hazard of glaucoma and the added likelihood of a pupil that dilates poorly and a zonule that is likely to disrupt easily. Also remember that the hypermature cataract is more likely to undergo spontaneous dislocation. These are cases to be avoided — at least to begin with.

It is of great help to know how well the pupil will dilate prior to the operation: test at the patient's outpatient visit. Then record whether dilation is full, three-quarters, half or very poor. A pupil that will not dilate to three-quarters should not be considered for an extracapsular extraction by the beginner. Many old people have rigid pupils. So also do patients who have been on miotics and patients with pseudoexfoliation. Such patients may have an extracapsular extraction but the technique of operation will have to be adjusted, as will be discussed later. Dilate at the outpatient visit to avoid possible pupillary fatigue that may be caused by using mydriatics within four days of the operation.

While the pupil is well dilated it is helpful to

examine the cataract. It is useful to know whether the nucleus of the cataract is hard or soft and how large it is. The age of the patient is the main indicator of nucleus size: the older the patient the larger the nucleus. The colour of the nucleus is the indicator of its hardness: clear, white, pale yellow, dark yellow, brown or red-brown and finally black — these colours indicate a progressive hardness of the nucleus. The size and hardness of the nucleus will affect one's size of incision and method of nucleus removal. Take this opportunity to examine for vitreous in the anterior chamber. It is advisable to detect this before the eye is opened.

The refractive history of the patient must be noted. The surgeon's interest in the refractive state will vary according to whether the patient has bilateral cataract, in which one is likely to plan for emmetropia, or a uniocular cataract where one may wish to aim for a planned degree of ametropia. One's interest will also vary according to the availability and accuracy of ultrasonic measurement. If such measurement is not available then a careful scrutiny of the past refractive history is vital, preferably from at least five years before. This is seldom directly available from the patient. Occasionally they may produce glasses dating to

a period prior to the onset of their cataract. The patient may have made an earlier visit to the hospital and the records may show an earlier refraction. All too often they do not. The patient's optician may hold early records and it is well worth the effort of communicating with him. All too often however the surgeon can obtain no previous record and he must then decide whether any myopia, most frequently met, is lenticular or axial. The patient's comment that the eye used to be all right is often misleading and if errors are to be avoided there is no alternative to accurate measurement. For the beginner therefore it is safer to start with patients with known refractive histories and not to gamble and possibly produce a minus eight or ten dioptre surprise.

Initial assessment should have detected any of the relative contraindications to the extracapsular method or have indicated any possible variations in the technique that might be necessary and whether the patient is to be operated on under local or general anaesthesia.

We shall now go on to consider the detailed preparation of the patient on his admission to hospital.

# 4

# Preparation

Once the patient has come into the ward specific preparation for the extracapsular method can begin. This will include keratometry, ultrascan and lens power calculation for emmetropia or ametropia if not already done in the outpatient department. Ideally the cornea should not be applanated immediately before operation for measurement of the pressure or for axial length measurement. Both procedures may affect subsequent corneal clarity.

Most of the ward preparation is directed towards dilation of the pupil. The surgeon will already have an accurate idea of the pupil's ability to dilate. It is necessary to co-operate fully with the ward sister and her staff. This is particularly required if extracapsular extractions are being done as a new procedure, as the ward staff will have less understanding of the problems involved than the surgeon. It is therefore up to him to talk to the ward staff. He must tell them about the advantages and difficulties of the operation, how vitally important it is to have a dilated pupil — a pupil that is fully dilated — and how without their help the operation will become much more difficult and the result for the patient may be compromised. The sister will rapidly learn what is meant by a dilated pupil — as one sister said to me, 'I began to get worried when I couldn't see the iris any more.' This approach may seem elementary but is a most rewarding one. Not only are those long frustrating minutes in theatre waiting for the pupil to dilate avoided but the added bonus of a greater postoperative awareness and interest from the ward staff is gained. All of this is to the patient's benefit.

I write specific instructions to instil the following drops into the eye every five minutes,

starting one hour before the estimated time of surgery and continuing until the patient leaves the ward: tropicamide 1%, phenylephrine 10%, cyclopentolate 0.5%.

If the patient is to have a local anaesthetic then some local anaesthetic drops will have to be used. All topical anaesthetic drops have an unfortunate clouding effect upon the corneal epithelium. This may affect observation through the cornea at a later stage of the procedure. This is another good reason for preferring general anaesthesia.

Prostaglandin inhibitors — indomethacin drops — are used preoperatively to reduce the subsequent level of prostaglandins released by stroking the iris. This will help to maintain a dilated pupil and may reduce postoperative iritis.

In the theatre there are further measures to help maintain the dilated pupil. More drops are instilled if necessary. Half a millilitre of bupivacaine hydrochloride 0.5% with hyaluronidase is given by retrobulbar injection — the long acting bupivacaine gives some postoperative analgesia as well. This injection is given in addition to any general anaesthetic. It blocks the parasympathetic nerve endings and prevents release of acetylcholine at the nerve endings, thus maintaining pupillary dilation. A small volume is used so as not to increase intraorbital pressure. If the operation is to be done under local anaesthetic the retrobulbar bupivacaine is mixed with adrenaline 1:200 000 and hyaluronidase 1500 units. Ten millilitres of the agent are used, 3 ml retrobulbar and the remainder for the eyelids, facial nerve blocks and 1 ml subconjunctivally.

A solution of 1:1000 adrenaline, as used for intracardiac injection, is added to the 500 ml container holding the infusion fluid. This helps to maintain pupillary dilation during the irrigation/aspiration. Ask your anaesthetist's consent before using it.

The second set of main preoperative measures are directed towards producing and maintaining a soft eye.

In order to operate safely within the anterior chamber it is essential to have enough space in which to carry out the necessary manipulations and manoeuvres. These manoeuvres include the anterior capsulotomy and the insertion of any type of lens implant. The longest procedure however is the aspiration and irrigation for removal of the residual cortex. The anterior capsulotomy can be done with a completely closed chamber, and the chamber can be maintained for a short period using any of the currently available viscous substances. However, the aspiration irrigation cannot be done in this way as the viscous substance would be aspirated immediately. It is possible to operate in a partly closed chamber but this cannot be relied upon if there is any tendency for the anterior chamber to collapse. Effective aspiration is difficult when trying to manoeuvre in such a chamber — especially at the twelve o'clock position. Most of the injury to the corneal endothelium therefore comes from attempting to manipulate in a shallow chamber. In many instances the anterior chamber remains deep throughout the procedure and there are no problems. It may therefore be thought that it is unnecessary to bother with steps to deepen it still further. Indeed you may be told that you will have difficulty removing the nucleus if the chamber is too deep. This is to some extent true, but is as nothing compared with the problems you will have attempting to finish the operation in an increasingly shallow chamber.

There will be some softening effect from the retrobulbar injection, especially if a full block is given. Nevertheless, the injection of 3 ml of fluid into the closed space of the orbit may significantly bulge the globe. Hence the necessity for the use of hyaluronidase and a little massage to ensure that the injected fluid diffuses throughout the orbital tissues.

The general anaesthetic reduces the ocular pressure still further, providing it is given smoothly and the patient's blood gas levels are maintained. Any straining or $CO_2$ retention will dramatically increase blood flow to the head and will produce a congested eye.

A period of sustained massage is the only satisfactory way to ensure that the ocular volume will be reduced and a deep anterior chamber will be maintained throughout the operation. Some form of 'balloon' is now the instrument of choice. A steady pressure of 35 mm Hg, readable on a dial, is applied to the orbit for a period of twenty minutes. This makes certain that the eye is soft. The chosen pressure level also ensures that undue pressure is not applied to the ocular circulation with possible ischaemic effects.

If a balloon is not available then digital massage is as effective, if rather tedious and not as exact. Two or three large swabs are doubled over and placed over the closed eyelid. Pressure is then applied, with the flat of the fingers, ten seconds on and five seconds off. This should be continued for twenty minutes. This sustained pressure, however produced, reduces the ocular and orbital volume. However, there is a rebound effect which seems to occur some twenty to thirty minutes after cessation of the pressure. This may not be quite long enough for you to finish the operation.

These procedures might seem to be unnecessary and also to add twenty minutes to the operation time. This is indeed a consideration. It is, however, absolutely necessary for the extracapsular operation to be successfully completed on every occasion. The patient can easily be brought to the theatre earlier than is customary with a little extra organization. The balloon is then applied in good time and any delay between cases is reduced to a minimum.

Lastly, the customary measures during the operation to reduce pressure on the globe from lid retraction sutures, a superior rectus suture and possibly a steridrape must be remembered.

The operation can now be begun with a soft eye and fully dilated pupil.

dropped onto the cornea. Don't imagine that you will be able to put on enough drops yourself. This will be impossible. A dripper connected to an infusion set and taped to the microscope can be readily adjusted for position and rate of flow to overcome this problem.

The next problem with visibility comes from the very fluid being used to keep the cornea clear. This collects in a pool, usually along the lower lid margin. The rising tide progressively cuts off the view, which becomes darker and darker. Your assistant's second task is therefore to mop up residual fluid. A little fluid can be mopped up with small sponges; larger amounts are better dealt with by opening out a large swab and using it as a wick. There is no great difficulty at this stage of the operation but later on during the irrigation there are larger volumes of fluid to be removed in a short space of time, which may be vital to the immediate task in hand. If no assistant is available a mechanical sucker can be used.

The remaining factors necessary for visibility involve the microscope. It is helpful to vary the magnification. The capsulotomy, for example, is best done with high magnification. The high power field is small and during the capsulotomy it will be necessary to centre and re-centre one's working area, using the X/Y shift. It is also usually necessary to adjust the fine focus as the capsule is seldom all in the same horizontal plane during the capsulotomy.

The third and final important factor is maintenance of the anterior chamber. The capsulotomy is done before the incision is completed, through a small stab incision. the anterior chamber is therefore completely closed. There will be some escape of aqueous on entering the chamber and occasionally during the subsequent manoeuvres. This may cause difficulty.

The needle may catch in the iris or be difficult to disengage from the capsule without endangering the cornea. It is better therefore to main-

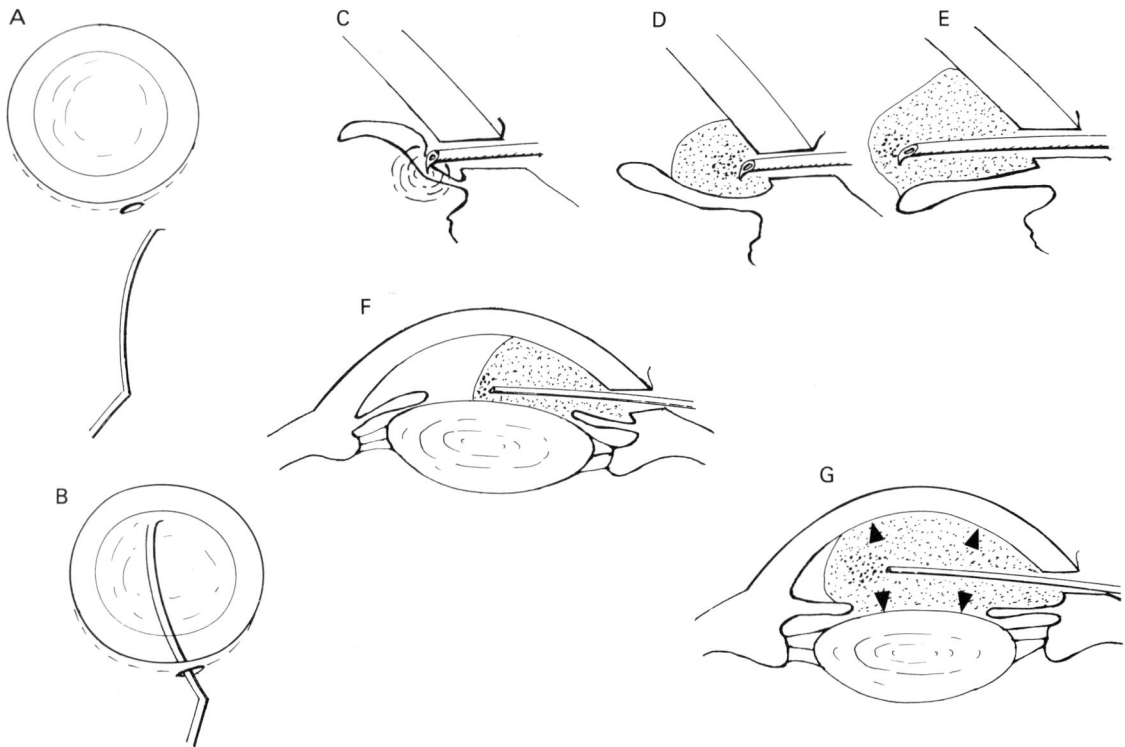

Fig. 5.1 Capsulotomy: **A** Insert capsulotomy needle, point horizontal **B** Advance to six o'clock **C, D, E** Inject Healon to free iris **F, G** Deepen anterior chamber with Healon

# 5

# Anterior capsulotomy

The essentials:
- a fully dilated pupil
- maximum visibility
- a deep anterior chamber.

The instruments required:
- 25 gauge irrigating cystitome
- Healon* and syringe
- fixation forceps.

The means of achieving maximum dilation of the pupil has already been described in some detail. It must now be maintained as far as possible. To do this the iris must not be stimulated by direct contact with the capsulotomy needle. It is easy to catch the edge of the iris on entering the anterior chamber or while attempting to make the capsulotomy as total as possible. One is therefore more likely to catch the iris if the pupil is not fully dilated to begin with. The pupil will also begin to constrict if the anterior chamber collapses — yet another reason for maintaining it.

You will soon find how easy it is for the surgeon's view to become obscured. If you can't see the capsule how can you cut it accurately? If you can't see clearly at the start of the operation, when everything is under control and in your favour, then how do you expect to be able to see a tear in the posterior capsule later on in the procedure?

It is therefore necessary to take steps throughout the procedure to retain maximum visibility. First, the eye should be positioned vertically so that the axial illumination from the microscope will be reflected from the fundus to produce a helpful red reflex against which the lenticular structures can be seen — the anterior capsule, cortex and particularly, as we shall see later, the posterior capsule. This red reflex will only be seen when the eye is vertical and when the pupil is dilated more than about 6 mm. If the pupil comes down, the red reflex is shut off and your view with it.

It may be difficult to position the eye correctly. The eyelids may be tight and the globe deep in the orbit both of which might make exposure for the incision difficult unless the eye is turned down. Similarly it may be difficult to extend the patient's neck sufficiently — in an old person or where there is arthritis, for example. It is worth your taking some time to position the patient's body, head and eye to achieve the best possible surgical exposure before beginning.

Once an excellent position has been achieved it is then mandatory to keep the cornea clear. The cornea rapidly dries out during the procedure, and as it is certainly going to take longer than an intracapsular extraction, and is liable to be affected by any casual instrumentation, by previously administered local anaesthetic drops and by the heat of the operating lamps, you must therefore keep the cornea constantly moist. A dedicated assistant, with constant hectoring, will drop fluid on to the cornea every 30 seconds. There are moments when he or she will be otherwise occupied or the fluid container will be emptied and a lapse of a minute or two will cause the cornea to opacify and remain so for the rest of the operation. If you use an assistant, make sure the fluid is in a 20 ml syringe — it is amazing how often there seems not to be a 20 ml syringe in the theatre — and make sure that the assistant's only task is to keep the cornea clear. If you have no assistant then you must use some automatic method to ensure that fluid is constantly

* Healon is the registered trademark of Pharmacia A.B.

tain the chamber positively. Air may be used for this purpose. Unfortunately, air has a tendency to pop out with a quick collapse of the anterior chamber. It may also be difficult to see through the bubble, particularly towards its edge. If the capsulotomy needle is attached to the irrigation set or to a fluid-filled syringe then the chamber may be refilled if there is any tendency to shallowing. This gives a good view but requires an extra manipulation just when you want to be concentrating on the capsule. I prefer to use a viscous substance, such as sodium hyaluronate, in every patient. The capsulotomy needle is attached to the syringe containing the viscous solution, which is convenient to hold.

The needle point is inserted into the anterior chamber and enough of the solution injected to push away the iris and maintain or deepen the chamber (Fig. 5.1). You then have total control of depth and perfect visibility through to the capsule.

The technique that I am going to describe is a simple one which only requires simple instruments — for the most part disposable. They are readily available.

The eye has, it is assumed, now been prepared, the incision of choice has been made and the anterior chamber has been filled with Healon and is ready for the capsulotomy.

An irrigating cystitome can readily be made from a disposable 25 gauge needle. I prefer the larger bore 25 gauge disposable cystitome, which gives a greater feeling of control and stability to movement.

This needle is now put into the anterior chamber. The hooked point is first positioned so that it will easily go through the small horizontal stab incision. This involves supinating one's hand (Fig. 5.1). Once the hook is through into the chamber a little Healon is injected.

The hook can then be advanced without fear of catching the iris. More Healon is injected. The hand can now be pronated so that the hook is pointing directly downwards towards the capsule. The needle is advanced to the six o'clock position (Fig. 5.2). It is placed just inside the pupil margin.

The projecting point is moved downwards into the capsule along the line of its axis. Usually a little dimple can be seen before it is penetrated.

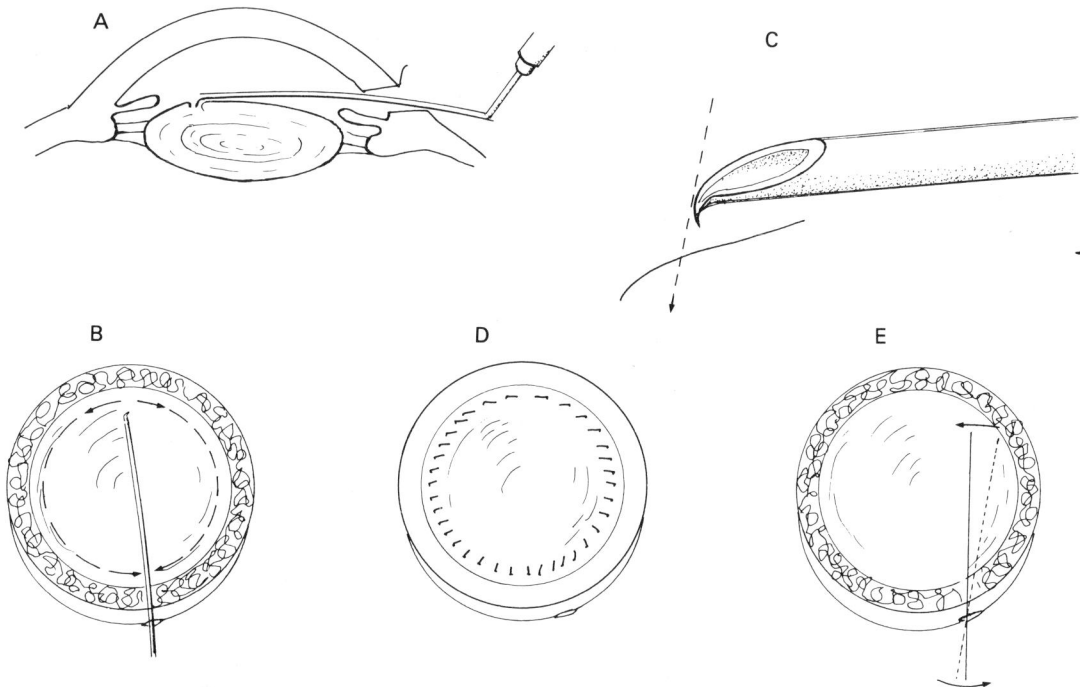

Fig. 5.2 Capsulotomy: **A, B** Position needle at six o'clock **C** Pierce capsule **D** Make 20–30 small cuts **E** Cut towards the pupil centre

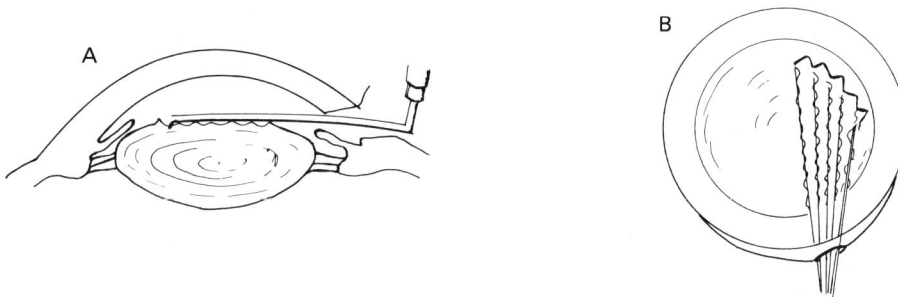

**Fig. 5.3** Capsulotomy: **A, B** Deep cuts or shallow AC disturb the cortex

Then with a little sideways rotation of the needle a short cut is made. It is not always easy to be sure that you have actually cut through the capsule, which may be surprisingly tough in young people. It may also be difficult to pierce where the contained cortex is soft or liquefied and there is no resistance to cut against, or if the disposable needle happens to be blunt.

If you press in too deeply, usually if the anterior chamber is shallow, you tend to disturb the cortex over the length of the needle (Fig. 5.3), which makes it harder to see the capsule. You can be sure you are through the capsule only when you see its cut edge or in a mature cataract when liquid cortical material gushes into the anterior chamber. Make this first cut small, less than 0.5 mm, and remember that the sharp edges of the needle will be engaged with side to side movements of the hand and not forward and backward movements. The first few cuts at the six o'clock position are therefore made tangential to the pupil.

The first cut having been successfully made, the needle is moved a little further round the capsule and the second cut made. Subsequent cuts are made around one side to the twelve o'clock position — about a dozen altogether. The needle is then returned to the six o'clock position and a similar number of cuts are made around the other side (Fig. 5.2). The cuts at three and nine o'clock will be exactly radial, directed towards the centre of the pupil. Towards twelve o'clock it becomes difficult to cut with a side to side movement because the length of needle within the eye is too short to pivot sufficiently. Cuts in this position are therefore made from the pupil margin away from you. Every cut should be separate and distinct and directed as far as possible away from the iris towards the centre of the pupil.

If a large cut is made or if the small cuts join together then a large flap of capsule is formed. It is then very easy to continue making the cuts beneath the capsule into the cortex without being aware that the capsule is uncut (Fig. 5.4). To avoid this you should lift the needle well out of the capsule between each cut. This has been likened to the action of rowing. The oar is

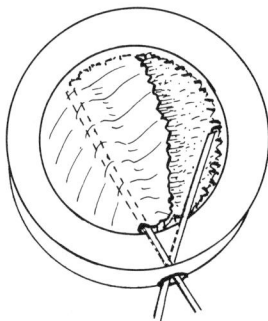

**Fig. 5.4** Capsulotomy: Needle advances beneath a capsular flap

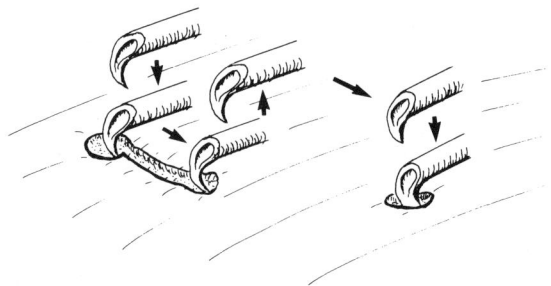

**Fig. 5.5** Capsulotomy: Cutting the capsule, likened to rowing a boat

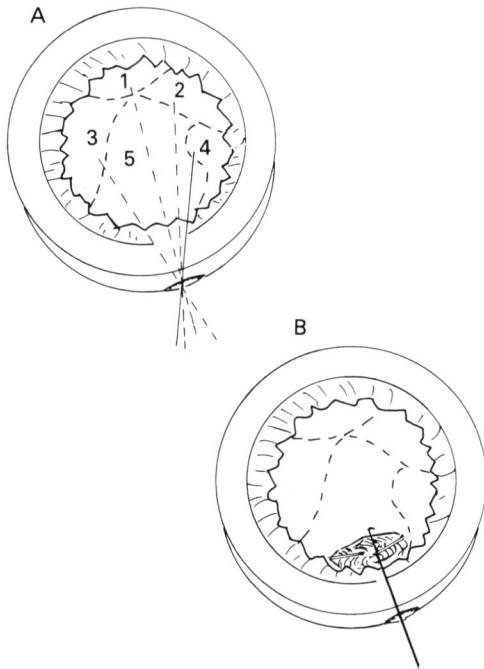

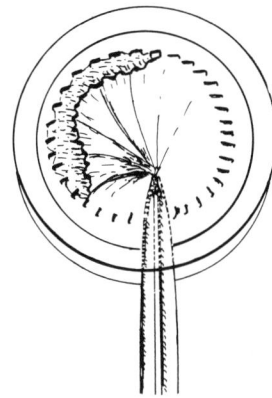

Fig. 5.7 Capsulotomy: 'Tear along the dotted line'

Fig. 5.6 Capsulotomy: **A, B** Scrape the capsule towards twelve o'clock

dropped into the water, the stroke made and the oar lifted clear of the water for the return stroke. It is then dropped into the water for the start of the next stroke (Fig. 5.5). Large flaps may cause difficulties later on and can be avoided at this stage if you are able to identify the cut edge of the capsule as you are making the capsulotomy.

Once you have completed the cuts you may scrape the loosened capsule into a heap in the centre of the lens (Fig. 5.6). This confirms that it is completely separated. Alternatively, once the incision has been completed, you may grasp the capsule in the centre with the fine plain forceps and remove the anterior capsule by 'tearing along the dotted line' (Fig. 5.7). It is better to do this than to hope that the capsule will be delivered along with the nucleus.

The technique that I use makes it necessary to remove all of the anterior capsule. I do not want any capsular tags, flaps or pockets. If these are unintentionally left behind then added difficulties will exist when the attempt is make to dislocate the nucleus and during aspiration of the cortex. Cortical material may remain trapped between the

two layers of the capsule or a capsular tag may block the aspiration port. It is then possible to pull on the capsule causing a tear or zonular dehiscence, both of which are to be avoided. So considerable care and attention should be given to the anterior capsulotomy if the subsequent stages of the procedure are not to become too difficult.

One's main difficulties come from a poorly dilated pupil or a pupil that constricts during the capsulotomy, along with the above mentioned factors which further obscure one's view. The beginner is strongly advised to start only on an eye where the pupil dilates fully. Once some experience has been gained various additional manoeuvres can be attempted to help you contend with a pupil that dilates poorly.

If the pupil dilates to three-quarters then it is possible to use the cystitome needle as an iris retractor, a one-handed technique: the side of the hooked portion retracts the iris immediately before the point is sunk into the capsule (Fig. 5.8). Healon can be injected beneath the iris margin. This will lift the iris enough to allow your cystitome to reach the peripheral capsule. A more certain method is to use a cystitome with a collar-stud attachment at the junction of the shaft and hook. This offers more certainty with the retraction. The iris is unlikely to slip off. This too is a one-handed method. Unfortunately this is not a disposable instrument and the sharpness is likely to diminish with repeated use. An alternative two-handed method makes use of a separate collar-stud retractor which is inserted through a separate stab

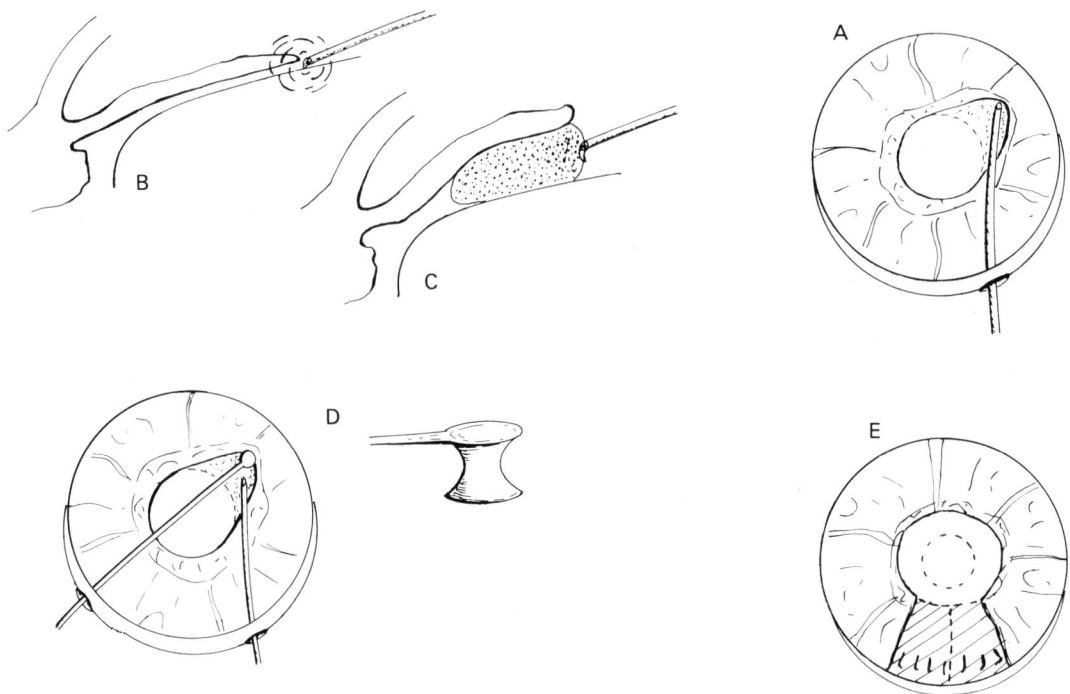

**Fig. 5.8** Capsulotomy: **A** Retract iris with capsulotomy needle **B, C** Lift iris with Healon **D** Retract iris with collar-stud — two-handed **E** Sector iridectomy

incision and manipulated by the other hand. This provides excellent iris retraction and may be used later on during aspiration of the cortex. Use of and co-ordination of the two hands does however require some practice before it becomes an easy technique.

Lastly, if the pupil will not dilate and an extra-capsular has to be done then a sector iridectomy may be done after completion of the section. The difficult twelve o'clock position can then be reached under direct vision with the cornea lifted. The iris is easily retracted to deal with the remainder of the capsule, the nucleus and cortex. A sector iridectomy is no bar to subsequent insertion of a posterior chamber lens.

Capsular tags or larger flaps at the twelve o'clock position can be removed with fine forceps and scissors. The edge of the tag is grasped, gently withdrawn with no tension put on the zonule, before it is cut off with de Wecker's or Vannas scissors. Flaps in this position make cortical aspiration particularly difficult and may also get caught in the wound if not seen and dealt with (Fig. 5.9). They are easier to remove than flaps at the six

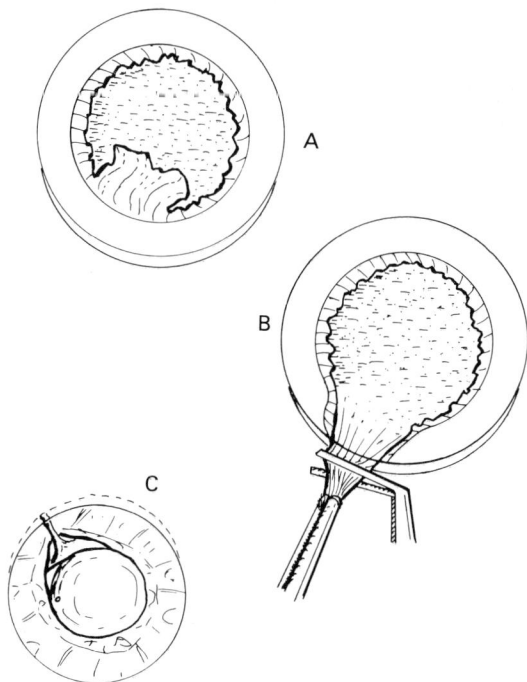

**Fig. 5.9** Capsulotomy: **A** Large flap of capsule at twelve o'clock **B** Abscissed with de Wecker's Scissors **C** Capsule incarcerated in incision

o'clock position or on either side, however. It is dangerous to pull on any broad-based flap — posterior capsule rupture or zonular dehiscence will occur. It is surprisingly difficult to traverse the anterior chamber with scissors and forceps, manoeuvre the anterior capsule away from the posterior capsule and cut it neatly. The anterior chamber is liable to collapse. You may injure the cornea or perforate the posterior capsule. At best one only manages to reduce the flap in size, because the flap moves away from the scissor blades as they close. The answer is to be sure to cut the capsule correctly at the six o'clock position at the beginning of the procedure. At this stage the capsule is tense and supported by the underlying cortex and is easiest to cut. Hence the advice to start the capsulotomy at six o'clock and not twelve o'clock. It is easier to tidy up at the top than at the bottom.

An anterior chamber which collapses is an occasional problem if continuous irrigation or air are used. The needle may then get trapped in the lens or iris. The anterior chamber must be reformed immediately, the needle disengaged and the capsulotomy continued. You will however have damaged the corneal endothelium and stimulated constriction of the iris. This will make everything more difficult later on. Therefore use Healon for all your patients. A collapsing anterior chamber is then virtually impossible and you will gain enormously in confidence. When you have gained more experience you may of course decide to modify this technique. Occasionally when doing a capsulotomy on a hypermature cataract the liquefied cortical material escapes from the capsular cut into the Healon-filled anterior chamber. It mixes with the Healon, completely obscuring the surgeon's view. This is annoying. If continuous irrigation is being used the material can easily be washed out. With Healon it will be necessary to wash out an expensive 0.5 ml of the viscous substance with balanced salt solution before refilling the anterior chamber with more Healon.

It is convenient to dislocate the nucleus before removing the cystitome from the eye and completing the incision, while the chamber is still closed, although I prefer to enlarge the incision and remove the anterior capsule before dislocating the nucleus. This and the subsequent removal of the nucleus will be dealt with in the next chapter.

A total or near total removal of the anterior capsule should have been achieved. The pupil should still be fully dilated and the surgeon's view of events crystal sharp. The nucleus should be dislocated and ready for removal. The incision must of course be completed and if necessary some preplaced sutures be put in. I only use preplaced sutures if difficulties are expected, as they do get in the way.

# 6

# Removal of the nucleus

The essentials:
— removal of the nucleus
— protection for the corneal endothelium
— maintenance of dilated pupil.

The instruments required:
— cystitome
— squint hook
— irrigating vectis
— corneal forceps
— Healon.

I again stress how important it is to maintain a dilated pupil. It is very easy to stimulate the iris during removal of the nucleus, often quite dramatically, so that the red reflex and the view of the cortex are severely interrupted. The corneal

endothelium is also at risk by direct damage from the hard nucleus and indirectly from instrumentation.

There are two methods of removing the nucleus. You may use the cystitome with expression or the irrigating vectis. It is necessary to be familiar with both methods as one or other may be more suitable in a particular situation.

The first manoeuvre, as was seen at the end of the chapter on the anterior capsulotomy, is dislocation of the superior pole of the nucleus into the anterior chamber. If the nucleus is hard, the usual indication being its colour, then it may be elevated using the irrigating cystitome (Fig. 6.1).

The hooked point is pushed into the edge of the nucleus at two o'clock. The nucleus is then

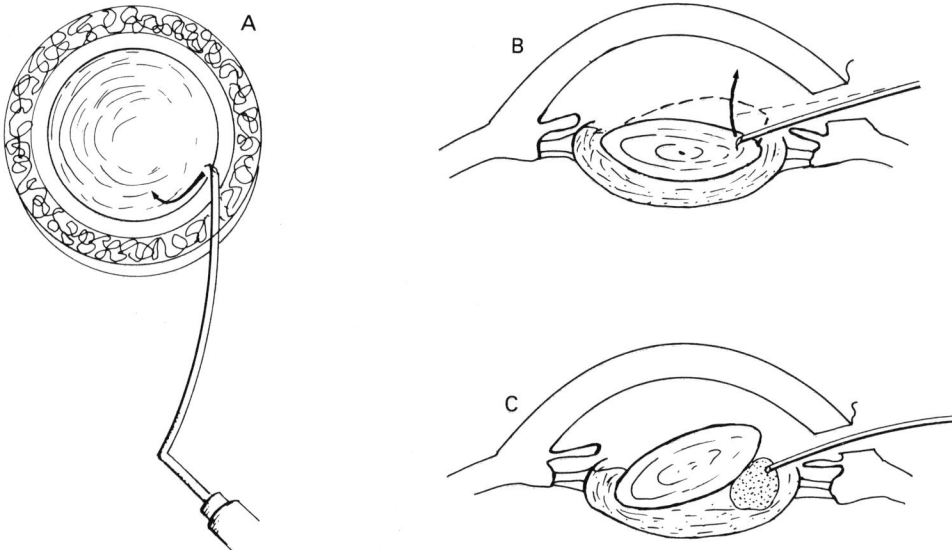

**Fig. 6.1** Nucleus: **A, B** Elevation and rotation with cystitome **C** Nucleus supported by Healon

16

rotated to the other side. If will be seen moving in relation to the peripheral part of the lens. Once it is moving freely then the cystitome is lifted forwards towards the cornea. If the cystitome starts to disengage from the nucleus then it may be pushed a little downwards at the same time as it is lifted towards the cornea. This should, if done successfully, bring the upper margin of the nucleus through the pupil into the anterior chamber. Sometimes there is a tendency for it to slip back behind the plane of the iris. Elevate it again. It should be well into the anterior chamber if the next part of the procedure is to be as simple as possible. Injection of a small amount of Healon beneath the upper pole of the nucleus will prevent it falling back into the posterior chamber.

If the nucleus is soft — clear, pale, or in a young person — it will probably fragment as you try to dislocate it with the cystitome. It is therefore better to use a different technique.

In this alternative method, a probe — a blunt tipped cannula, an iris repositor or cyclodialysis spatula is then moved across the pupil, towards cortex and nucleus in a position to one or other side of the twelve o'clock position (Fig. 6.2). The spatula is them moved across the pupil, towards the centre, separating and lifting the nucleus forwards from the posterior cortex. This method

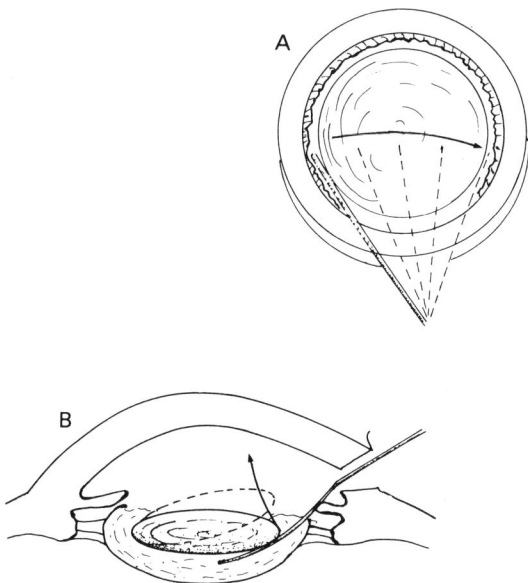

Fig. 6.2 A, B Elevation by 'tyre lever'

is likened to the manner in which a tyre lever is operated. This second method is better done after the incision has been completed. There is then more room to reach the ten or two o'clock positions at which the spatula is inserted. At first it may be difficult to find the right level and you may fear that your spatula will go through the posterior capsule. There is generally plenty of room. Remember the lens is more convex on its posterior aspect.

Using either method the nucleus should now be partly dislocated into the anterior chamber. If the cystitome method was used the incision will now be completed before the next step — removal of the nucleus.

Imagine that you have an elderly patient with a large, dark brown, hard nucleus. Your assistant will first lift the corneal rim a little. You will then hold the cystitome in your right hand with the hook directed to your left. In your left hand you will hold the expressing instrument of your choice; I use a squint hook. Apply it about 6–8 mm behind the wound edge, that is at the top of the eye and not on the lower sclera or cornea (Fig. 6.3). Gentle pressure will make the wound gape a little. Maintain enough pressure so that you can see the edge of the nucleus at the upper part of the anterior chamber. Make sure that your squint hook does not slip forwards on to the iris during the manoeuvre. Having achieved this position hold it steady while you move the hook of the cystitome into the edge of the nucleus; try and make sure that you have got a firm grip on it. Then move the cystitome to the left and towards you, thereby lifting the nucleus out of the eye. If the cystitome is not firmly planted in the nucleus it will detach itself and if the nucleus is soft or friable the point may break out. In either instance reinsert the cystitome towards the right-hand side and repeat the whole movement. Release your squint hook as the nucleus comes through the incision and let your assistant release the corneal flap. If the pupil is fully dilated, and the nucleus dislocated well forward, removal is possible with the cystitome alone, without expression (Fig. 6.4).

The main difficulties occur when the nucleus is small, soft or not well dislocated into the anterior chamber. You then find that the limited degree of

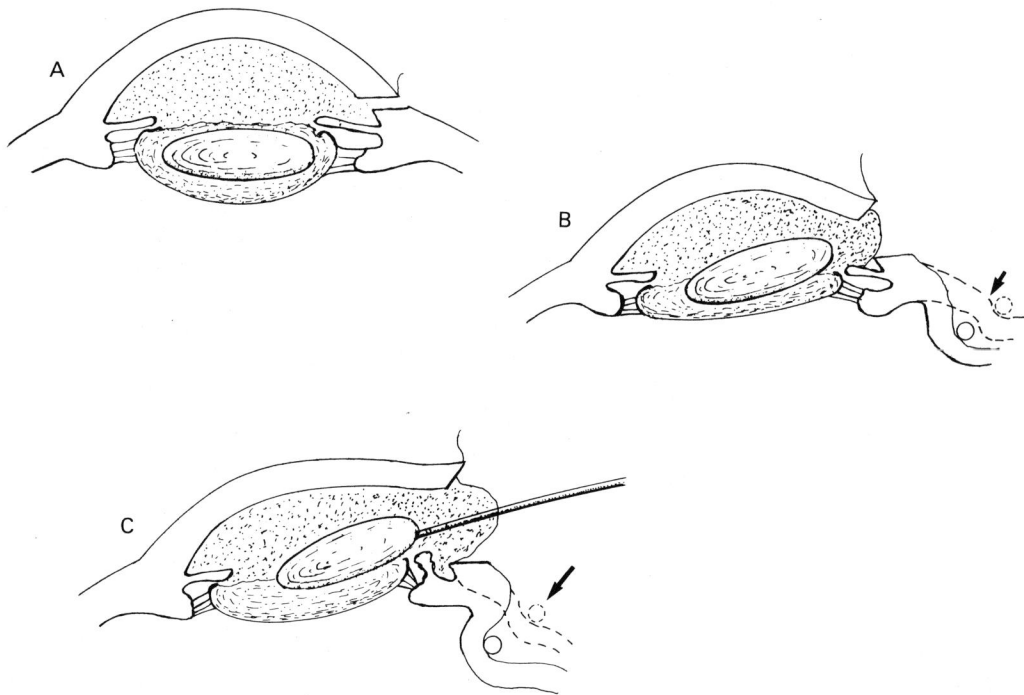

**Fig. 6.3** Nucleus: **A** Deep lying nucleus **B** Elevated by expression **C** Hooked out with cystitome

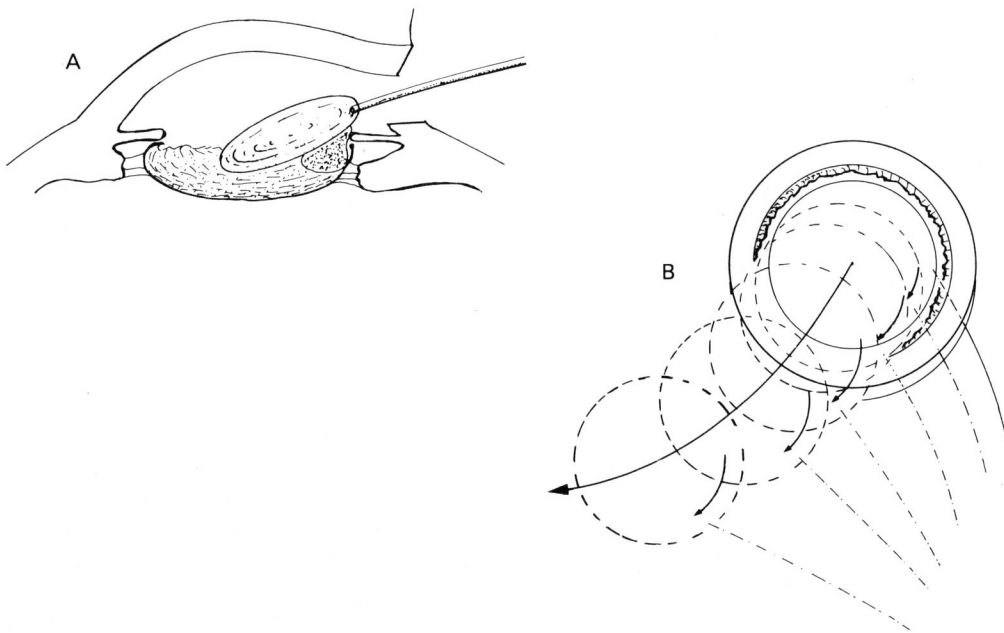

**Fig. 6.4** Nucleus: **A** Elevated nucleus supported by Healon **B** Wheeled out by cystitome without expression

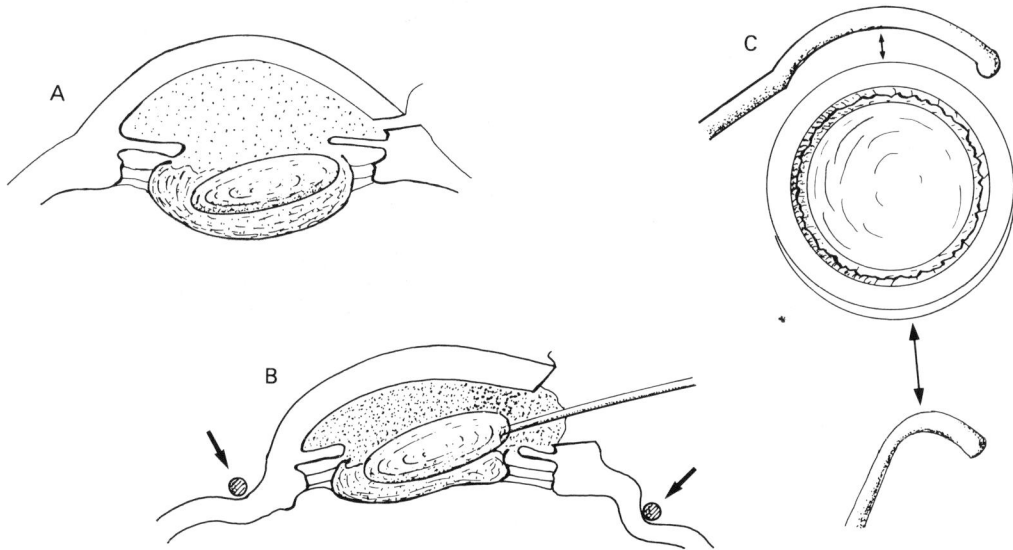

**Fig. 6.5** Nucleus: **A** Deep lying nucleus **B** Double expression **C** Position for expression

expression as described above is not enough to present the nucleus to your waiting cystitome or that pieces break off the nucleus leaving its main body behind. If you persist with expression you will then require a greater expressive force, still at the top position, but amplified by expression on the corneoscleral rim below (Fig. 6.5). This lower point of expression helps to dislocate the upper pole of the lens further into the anterior chamber. You may then proceed as before. However, the greater degree of expression used will almost certainly have a disastrous constricting effect on the pupil, which may contract by 3 mm in a few seconds. In addition expression over the lower

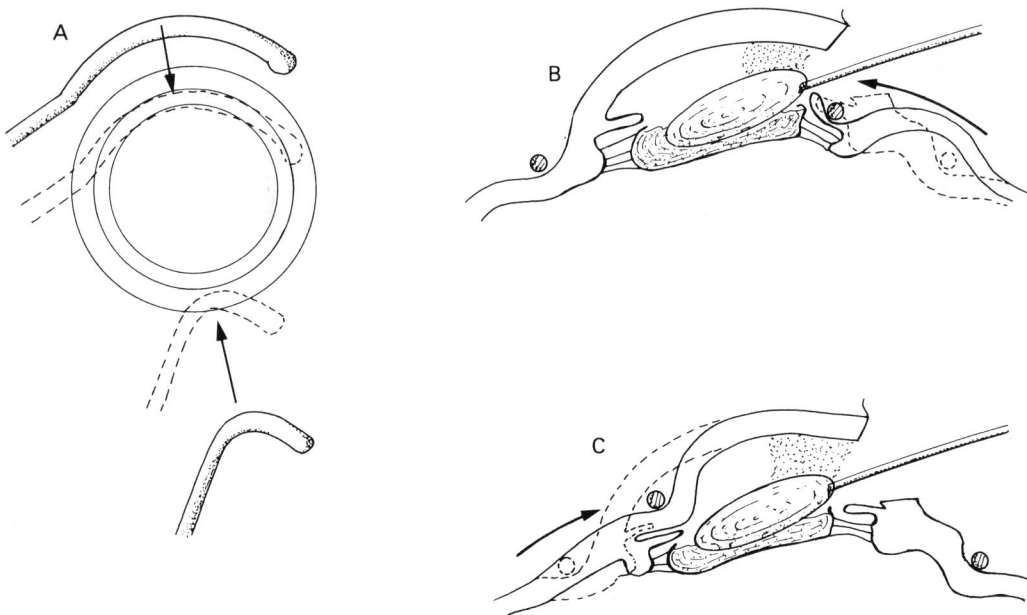

**Fig. 6.6** Nucleus: **A, B** Upper expressor slips onto iris **A, C** Lower expressor slips onto cornea

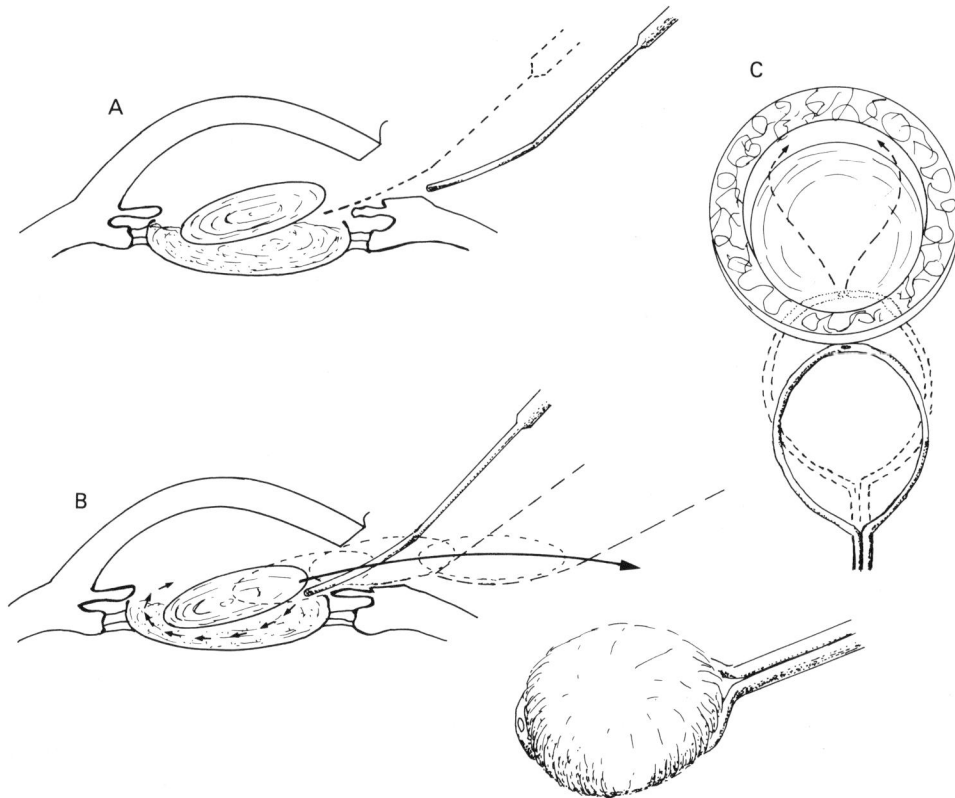

**Fig. 6.7** Nucleus: A Position and angle of vectis B, C Nucleus washed out by fluid pressure

corneosclera nearly always strays upwards on to the cornea itself, as you try to hold the nucleus upwards, so that direct damage occurs to the corneal endothelium — partly by bending the cornea and partly by rubbing the endothelium against the hard material of the nucleus (Fig. 6.6). These difficulties are avoided if the nucleus has been adequately dislocated and if the correct method has been chosen.

It is unlikely that problems would have occurred with a large hard nucleus, as described. Imagine now that you have a younger patient with a post traumatic cataract. The nucleus is small and soft. Once the nucleus has been elevated using the tyre lever method then the irrigating vectis, with either one or more holes, is attached to a 2 ml syringe containing balanced salt solution or Healon (Fig. 6.7). This is held in the right hand so that the open part of the vectis faces forwards and the irrigating hole is just behind the incision. The syringe and its plunger should be comfortably grasped so that fluid can easily be ejected in a controlled way. The end of the vectis is a long way from one's fingers at the top end of the syringe, which makes the whole instrument a little unwieldy. Practise a few times until it feels comfortable. The assistant again lifts the cornea just enough. The lower rim of the vectis is applied to the sclera just above the wound so that a little expression can be applied if the nucleus is not clearly visible. When it is visible the vectis is slid under the nucleus, the instrument following the posterior curve of the lens. Once the tip is behind the edge of the nucleus then you may start slowly injecting. It is often not necessary to insert the vectis any further. The stream of fluid directed between the nucleus and posterior capsule will wash the nucleus up and out of the eye. The open loop of the vectis merely serves to support it and finally withdraw it from the eye. The vectis is not used to lift the nucleus out of the eye.

The main difficulty in using the vectis is over-

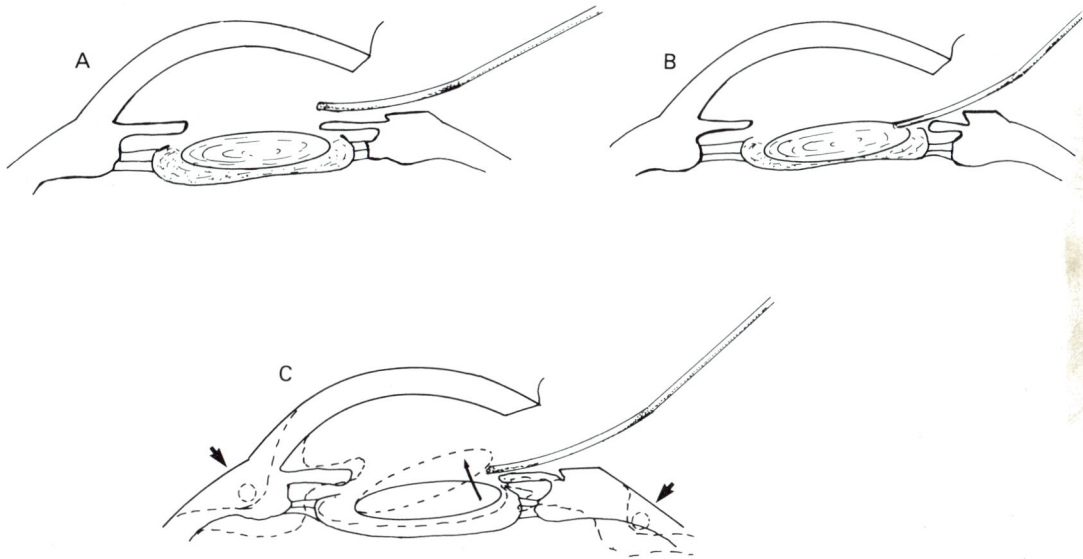

**Fig. 6.8** Nucleus: **A** Pupil constricted and nucleus not elevated **B** Vectis engaged anterior to equator of nucleus **C** Elevate nucleus prior to engaging the vectis

come if its mechanism is understood. Sometimes it may be difficult to engage the end of the vectis beneath the nucleus (Fig. 6.8). This may occur when the pupil constricts or when the nucleus has not been adequately elevated. Incorrect application of the vectis may directly stimulate the iris at the twelve o'clock position further constricting it. Occasionally it may be inserted through instead of under a very soft nucleus. Most of the nucleus is then left in the eye.

Further protection is given to the corneal endothelium throughout the removal of the nucleus by the use of Healon. You will recall that the anterior chamber was filled with Healon for the capsulo-

tomy (Figs 6.5, 6.6). This Healon remains within the eye, keeping a deep anterior chamber during dislocation of the nucleus and its subsequent removal by the cystitome or vectis. It makes a wonderful cushion to express against and helps to protect the endothelium both from direct instrumental injury and from injury from a hard nucleus. Healon is vastly superior to air, which is unpredictable, or watery solutions.

The second stage of the operation is now complete and a crystal clear cornea, a fully dilated pupil and a fully maintained anterior chamber still exist. Now we are prepared for the next stage of the operation — removal of the residual cortex.

# 7

# Removal of the cortex

The essentials:
- — removal of all the cortex
- — an intact posterior capsule
- — protection of the endothelium.

The instruments required:
- — irrigating cannulae — single and double/ coaxial irrigating aspirating (0.2, 0.3 and 0.6 mm)
- — iris retractor
- — capsule polishers
- — irrigating fluid.

The first essential is that all of the cortex is removed. Cortical material is irritating to the eye and will excite an immunological reaction — an acute iritis. This will lead to all sorts of problems, posterior synechiae between the iris and pseudophakos, an occluded pupil, peripheral anterior synechiae and secondary glaucoma. Iritis may also have an effect on the corneal endothelium and possibly promote cystoid macular oedema. It is of course impossible to remove all of the cortex, but every effort should be made to remove as much as possible, within the other essentials of the procedure. The factors which have most effect upon your ability to remove the cortex have been fully documented above — a fully dilated pupil, complete removal of the anterior capsule and continued visibility, this last being the result of a clear cornea, dilated pupil and correct use of the microscope.

It is obviously necessary to keep the posterior capsule intact. If we tear the posterior capsule we have immediately lost the advantages of the extracapsular method that we are striving for. This to some extent also includes the small controlled intentional posterior capsulotomy that is occasionally

necessary. For the beginner identification of the posterior capsule is probably the hardest task of the whole operation. Ideal conditions should be pursued to begin with so that this difficult observation is made as easy as possible. Clear visibility and coaxial illumination achieved through a dilated pupil and a crystal cornea produce the red reflex against which the filmy posterior capsule can be identified. Having identified the capsule it is a great help to maintain it in the same plane by maintaining the depth of the anterior chamber. It is kept intact by using all your instruments under direct visual control — as we shall see.

Removal of the cortex is the longest part of the operation and there is therefore more opportunity for you to damage the corneal endothelium. It must be protected from direct contact with your instruments. The central cornea is likely to be touched when the anterior chamber becomes shallow, due to vitreous pressure or when it collapses due to your aspirating faster than you are irrigating, or if you are particularly clumsy (Fig. 7.1). Vitreous pressure should have been prevented by your earlier manoeuvres to soften the eye. If vitreous pressure becomes troublesome make sure there is no external pressure on the globe. Then insert two or more sutures to close the anterior chamber partially. Increase the irrigating pressure until a deep chamber can be maintained and then continue.

The peripheral cornea, closest to the incision, is more prone to injury by instrumental contact. Make sure that you lift the edge of the cornea each time that you insert any instrument and try to reduce the number of instrumental insertions to the minimum. Angle your instruments so that no undue force is applied to the corneal edge. This

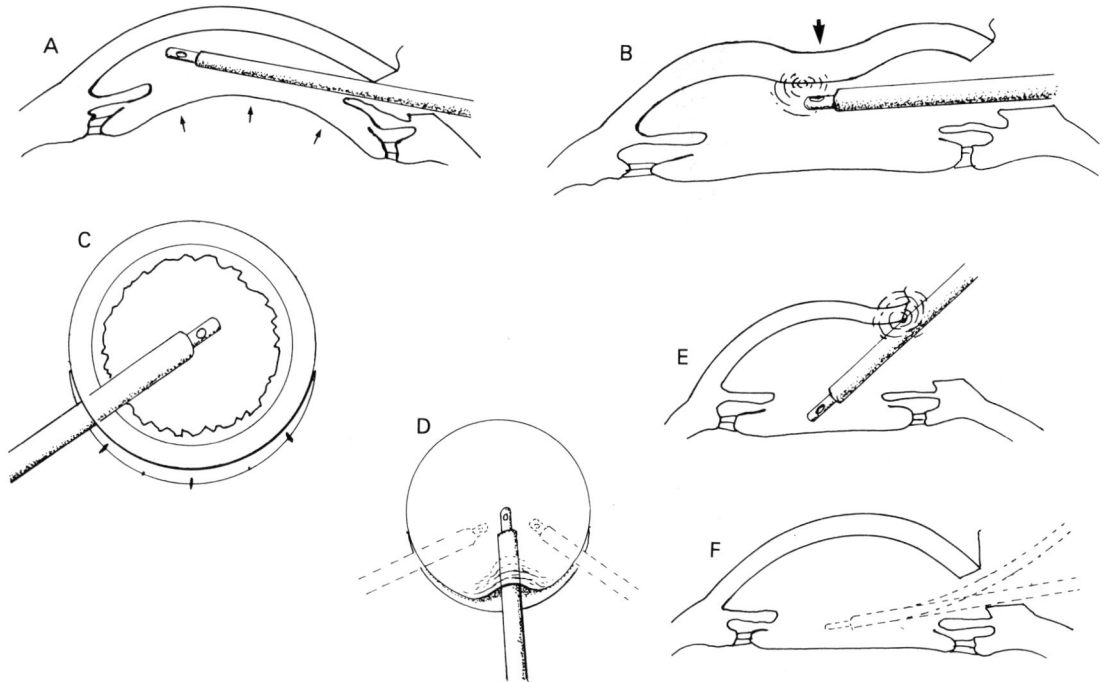

**Fig. 7.1** Cortex: **A** Shallow AC from vitreous pressure **B** AC collapses, aspiration too fast **C** Incision partially closed, increase irrigation reduce aspiration **D, E, F** Injury to peripheral cornea

may be difficult with a deep set eye or where exposure is poor. Check these points. Try to obtain instruments that are curved to make their insertion as easy as possible. Some protection may be offered to the peripheral cornea by using a small limbal-based flap which turns under the edge of the cornea or by bevelling the incision so that most of the instrumental contact occurs on the outer half of the corneal thickness. If you are able to complete the removal of the cortex through a completely open incision you will have much more room to manipulate your various cannulae to the most advantageous angle, both to remove cortex and to avoid corneal damage.

Some of the essentials have now been considered. Imagine first a mature or hypermature cataract. Conditions are ideal — the nucleus has been removed, the pupil is fully dilated and there is a deep stable anterior chamber. A shallow curved, blunt tipped cannula is attached to the infusion of warmed Hartmann's solution. It is held in the right hand so that the rate of flow can be controlled by digital pressure on the rubber bulb at the end of the tube. This provides a slightly flexible grasp to the needle, but it gives good control of the tip of the cannula. The cornea is lifted a little by forceps held in the left hand and the cannula inserted a little way. Irrigation is started (Fig. 7.2). Any loose material is readily washed away. The assistant mops up the excess fluid that collects in the conjunctival sac. The cannula is directed so that the fluid flows just below the level of the iris down towards the three o'clock position. The fluid takes a semicircular route, down one side and up the other — separating and washing out loose cortex. The cannula can be can be directed from one side of the incision along the upper margin of the iris so that cortex at the twelve o'clock position is reached. With the cortex already liquefied all of it may be removed by simple irrigation. Do this if it is possible. A single irrigating needle is smaller and less traumatic than the double cannulae and therefore preferable. Suitably curved or J-shaped cannulae may be used to wash away loose cortex not already removed. Inspect the posterior capsule, especially in the central area.

If there is residual cortex polish it away, as will

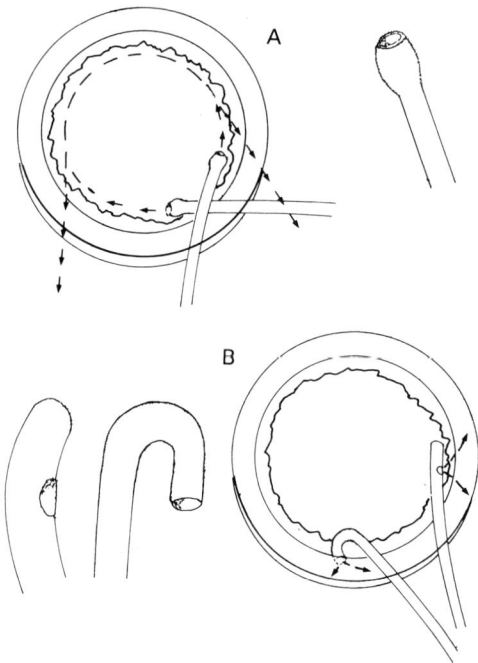

**Fig. 7.2** Cortex: **A** Straight irrigation **B** Curved and J-shaped irrigators

be described below. If the capsule is opaque a capsulotomy will be necessary. Most extractions for this type of cataract are completed without either of these manoeuvres. The eye would now be ready for a lens implant.

The procedure for an immature cataract will now be discussed. All or part of the cortex will be clear and the lens fibres normally formed. Their texture may vary from soft to moderately tough. Any loose cortex in the anterior chamber may be irrigated away as described above. It saves time and instrumental insertions to go straight to the coaxial irrigating/aspirating cannula (Fig. 7.3). The cannula is attached to the infusion tube on one side. the reservoir is raised to give a good pressure level and adjusted by the screw control which is positioned close to the cannula and thereby under the surgeon's control. A 10 ml syringe is attached — in a straight line — to the central needle of the double cannula. A coil spring is first placed between the handle of the plunger and the body of the syringe. The irrigation is now set to a steady drip rate, the assistant prepares to

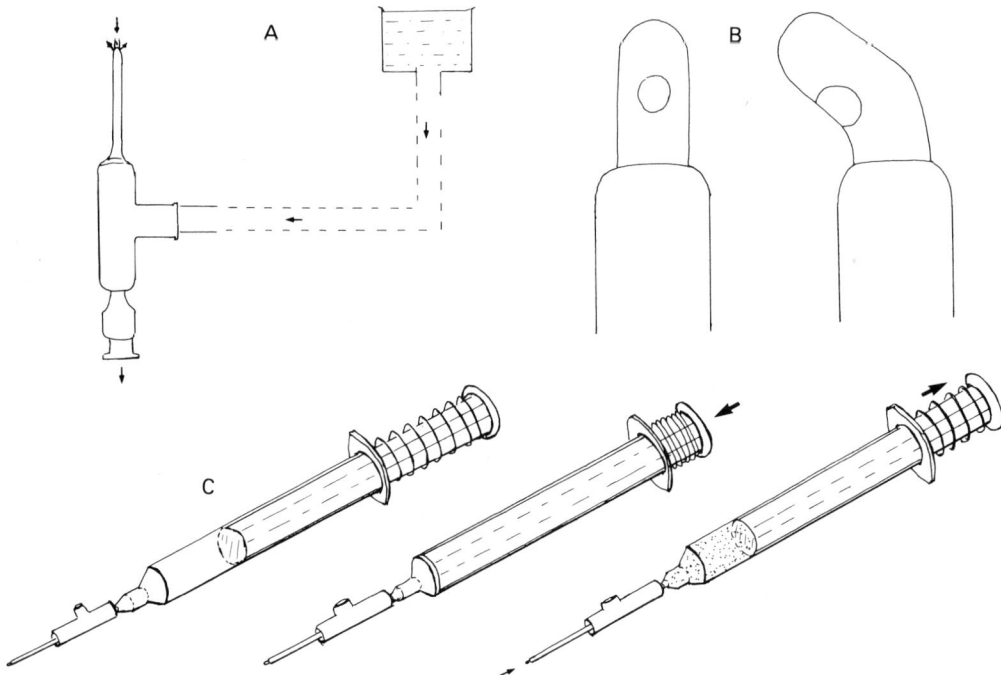

**Fig. 7.3** Cortex: **A** Aspiration/irrigation system **B** Needle tips **C** Spring loaded syringe for one-handed operation

mop and the syringe is emptied of air by compressing the coil spring and plunger. The aspiration port is identified and positioned in an upwards direction. The syringe is thus manipulated solely by the right hand. The irrigation is constant, but can be varied if necessary.

Aspiration is started by gently releasing the right thumb which is on the end of the plunger. The spring then moves the plunger. This may seem to be clumsy to begin with. The distance between your hand at the top of the syringe and the tip of the cannula is quite long and therefore control of the tip is not very direct or immediate. This must be learned by practice. The main advantage is that the left hand is thereby freed for other tasks. Its important tasks are to lift the cornea for introduction of the cannula and the possible operation of a second instrument within the anterior chamber — an iris retractor. Once the cannula is within the eye then the left hand can be used to support the lower end of the cannula. Further difficulties arise when trying to manoeuvre the cannula from side to side. The irrigating tube comes into the cannula at right angles and it is usually necessary for the assistant to support the trailing tube and follow you around.

You are now ready to begin. Position the aspiration port in the centre of the pupil, centre the microscope, adjust the magnification and focus. Begin by gently releasing your thumb on the plunger and watch the loose cortex closest to the port (Fig. 7.4). It will be drawn into the opening and after a short pause it will be sucked in and away. Maintain pressure on the plunger. If you release it suddenly or try to produce a greater suction power you will collapse the cornea on to your cannula. Move the tip of the cannula around the central area, gradually ingesting the looser bits of cortex. If all goes well you are now likely to be left with a ring of fairly obvious cortex protruding from under the edge of the iris and a variable amount of cortex, often quite clear, extending right across the posterior capsule.

Now move the tip of the cannula towards the six o'clock position just under the edge of the iris margin (Fig. 7.5). Try to keep it in view. Aspirate gently until you see that cortex has been drawn into the port. Stop aspirating, but don't release the suction, and draw the cannula towards the

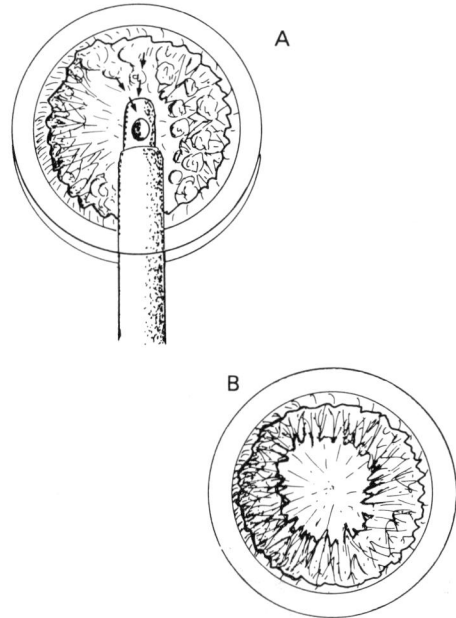

**Fig. 7.4** Cortex: **A** Aspiration of loose cortex **B** Residual adherent cortex

centre of the pupil. You will see that peripheral cortex is being drawn out from beneath the iris towards the centre of the anterior chamber. Draw it as far as you can, until the cannula is about to leave the eye or until the fragment of cortex has separated completely (Fig. 7.6). It usually has a triangular outline, broadest at the periphery and narrowing to a point towards the centre of the pupil — following the normal pattern of distribution of the lens fibres. You are now stripping the cortex. On either side of the triangular wedge that you have removed you will be able to see the edge of the neighbouring clear cortical fibres, between which will be a clear gap. This apparently structureless area is floored by the posterior capsule.

If the fragment is quite free then ingest it by gently releasing pressure on the plunger. If the fragment is still attached and the cannula is about to come out of the eye then slowly ingest part of the fragment of cortex, moving the tip of the cannula back towards its original position, in this instance at six o'clock. When you are there stop aspirating and strip again. The fragment should come free. Sometimes a little side to side movement will help to free it.

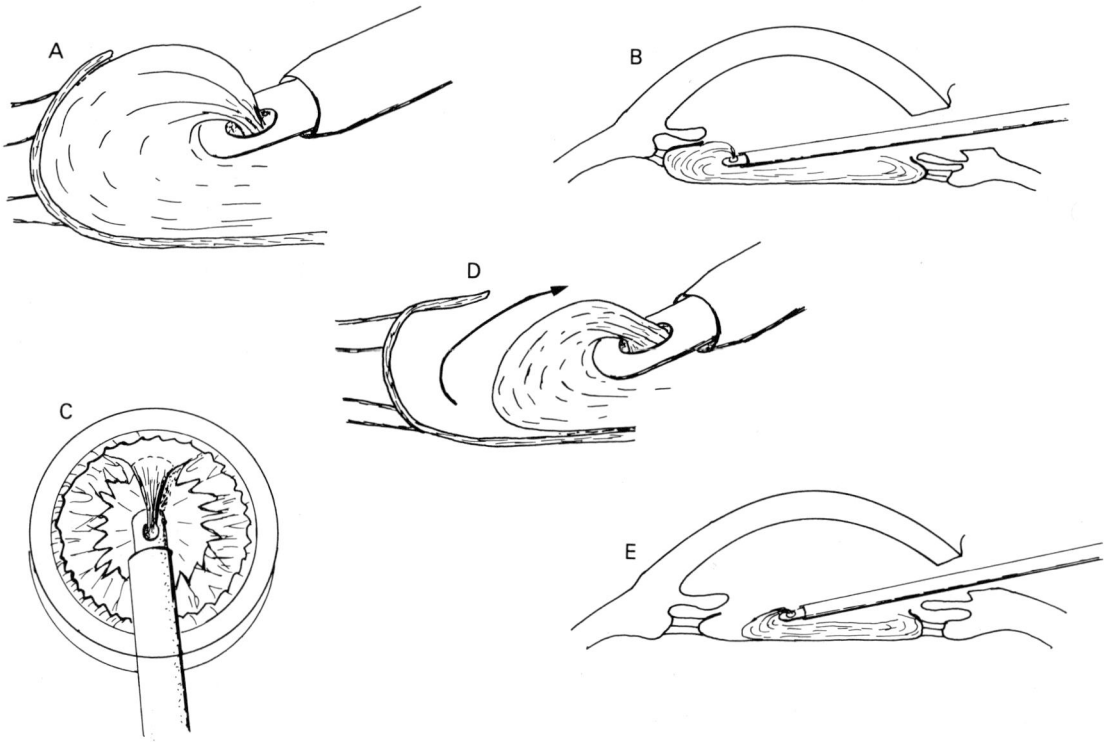

**Fig. 7.5** Cortex: **A, B, C** Six o'clock cortex drawn into aspirator **D, E** Cortex stripped towards pupil centre

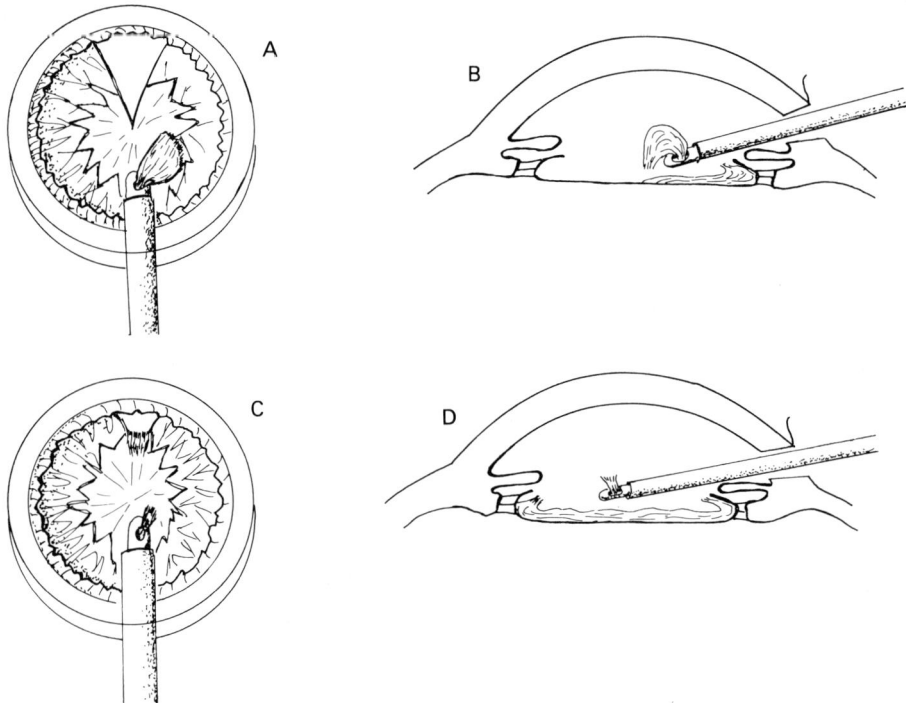

**Fig. 7.6** Cortex: **A, B** Triangular fragment stripped clear from capsule **C, D** Cortex broken off short

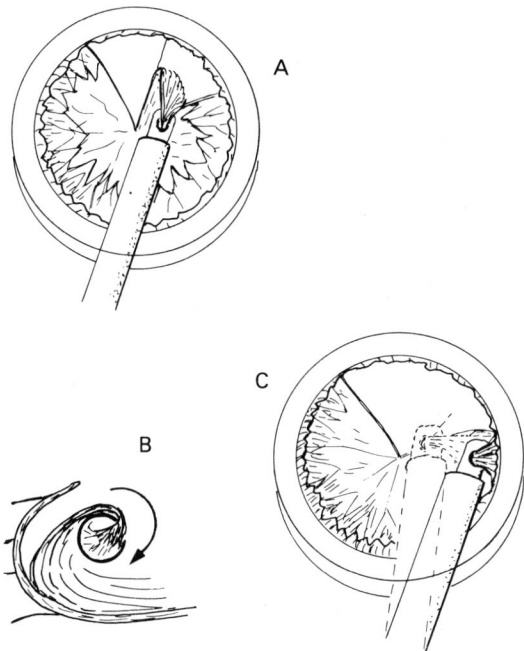

**Fig. 7.7** Cortex: **A** Strip cortex **B, C** Use a rotary movement at the sides

If you try to ingest the whole of the fragment before it is freed then it will break, leaving part of it on the central capsule or underneath the iris (Fig. 7.6). It is then harder to pick up again.

Now go to one or other side of the six o'clock position and repeat the procedure, each time stripping towards the centre. Sometimes a little rotary movement — about the long axis of your cannula — will help to pull cortical material out from beneath the iris (Fig. 7.7). But remember to keep the aspiration port in view and facing upwards all the time. Don't aspirate while the cannula tip is under the iris.

The rotary movement is specially useful for stripping cortical material down either side. Otherwise the whole cannula has to be moved or levered across from the iris margin towards the other side. This is an awkward movement to perform. Once the side are free then you have only the top to do.

It may be possible to go straight in from above and grasp cortex in the aspiration port while the

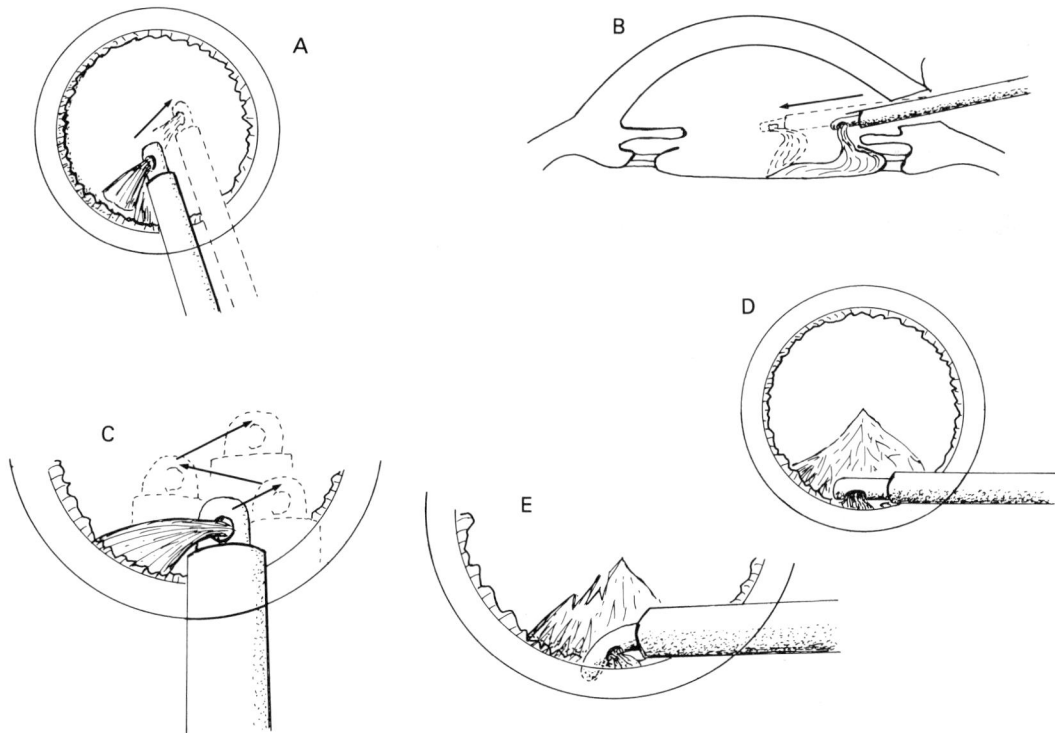

**Fig. 7.8** Cortex: **A, B** 'Over the top' for cortex at twelve o'clock **C** Work the cortex out **D** Introduce the A/I needle for the side **E** Curved I/A needle

cannula tip is still anterior to the plane of the iris (Fig. 7.8). Usually this fails and you must angle the cannula in, most easily from the temporal side of the incision so that the tip of the cannula can be brought below the pupil margin; i.e., posterior to it. Cortex is caught in the port and the cannula rotated between your fingers, so that the port turns upwards and away from you. Alternatively the double cannula with the curved tip may be used. This is easier than trying to move the end of the cannula towards the pupil centre.

You will now have removed most of the cortical fibres, though there may be a few wispy strands still protruding from beneath the iris and bits on the posterior capsule. The wispy strands are always attached to larger clumps of cortex — still hidden behind the iris. They can be drawn into the cannula port, but are often too small to be caught, so that when you try to strip them they just come out of the port. Try the smaller aspirating needle with an opening of 0.2 or 0.3 mm. If this fails then try polishing as described below.

Occasionally there will be obvious, or not so obvious, clear fibres on the posterior capsule, often left behind during stripping, or sometimes obvious fragments at the periphery. You will already have tried to remove the latter and be afraid to attempt the former, in case you break the capsule.

Both remnants can be freed using a polisher (Fig. 7.9). I always use the fine polisher attached to a syringe containing balanced salt solution. The peripheral fragments can readily be stirred around, loosening them and often leaving a portion that can then be readily aspirated. If these peripheral remnants still defy your efforts to remove them then leave them. It is better to be able to continue with an intact posterior capsule rather than worry over some residual lens material.

Small fragments on the more central part of the capsule should be gently rubbed with the fine polisher. Polish from clear capsule to fragment until you have elevated enough material to grasp

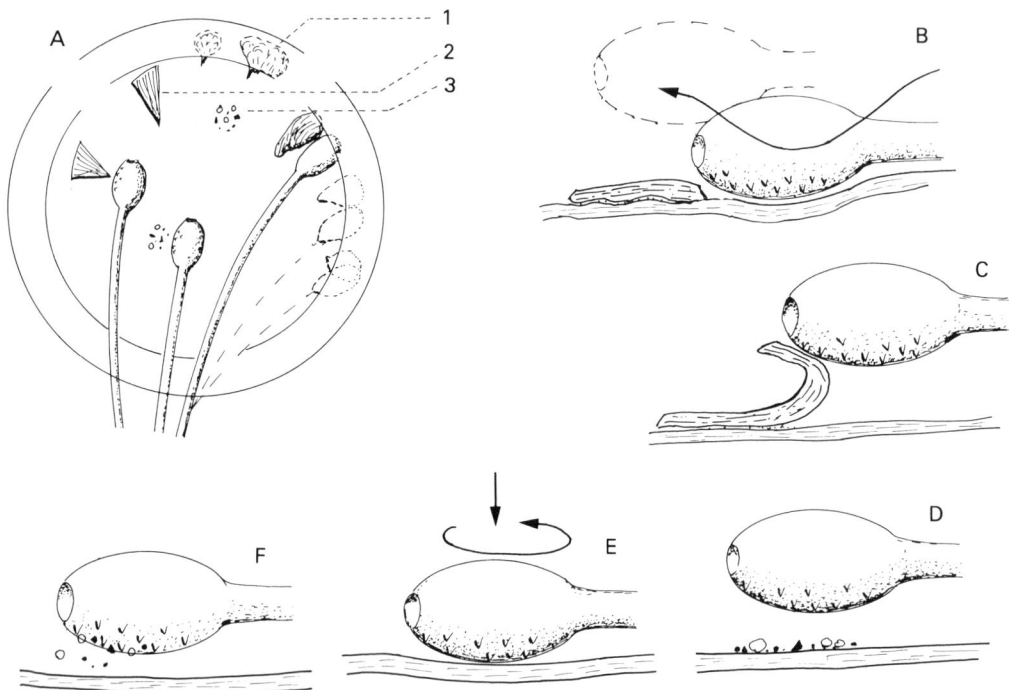

**Fig. 7.9** Polishing: **A** 1. Peripheral cortex 2. Flat plaques 3. Small fragments **B, C** Elevate edge of flat plaque **D, E, F** Circular polish for fragments

with your small aspiration needle. Remember to keep the port in view so that you don't aspirate the capsule. Sometimes gentle irrigation/aspiration with your small syringe through the polishing needle will help to clear the material and improve your view.

Finally inspect the capsule under high magnification, especially in the central area, for isolated spots of cortex. These can often be seen over quite a wide area and should be removed with further polishing. Use a circular rubbing or polishing motion. You will be able to see the fibres coming off; some can be irrigated away, some stick to the polisher and some will require more polishing (Fig. 7.9).

These manoeuvres presuppose that you can identify the posterior capsule. This is not always as easy as it is sometimes made out to be.

The conditions are now deal — coaxial illumination on the microscope, with the patient's eye looking vertically upwards. The cornea has been kept crystal clear by the assistant or the automatic dripper and the pupil is still fully dilated. There is now an excellent red reflex in the pupil.

We have also been able to maintain a soft eye with a deep anterior chamber — so we know that the posterior capsule will be lying in a plane well behind that of the iris. After centring the field of view, focus down to the iris, zoom up in magnification and begin looking for the tell-tale signs. During stripping of the cortex the capsule position should already have been noted. First of all look for obvious residual lens fibres in the centre of pupil — don't make the mistake of thinking that clear lens fibres are the capsule. Focus on these and increase the magnification. You may now see little fragments of fibres, sometimes short rod-like particles and sometimes round particles. These are *on* the capsule. Occasionally there may be a fibrotic plaque *in* the capsule, but remember that the capsule is one of the so-called glass membranes of the eye and therefore structureless at the microscopic level. You therefore cannot see it! What you can see are fragments on it and reflections coming off it (Fig. 7.10). During the stripping and polishing look for these reflections. When the capsule is moved, particularly when it is depressed or indented, the deformation causes the capsule to act like a concave mirror.

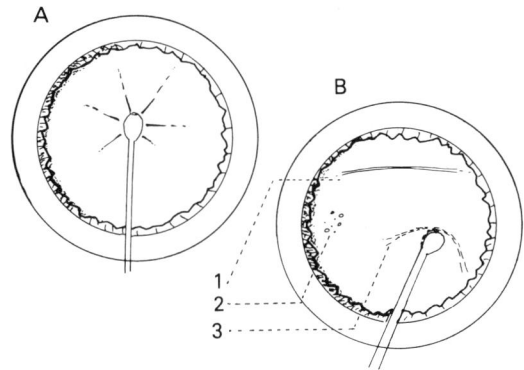

Fig. 7.10 Capsule: **A** Capsular reflections **B** 1. Tension lines from zonule 2. Spots on the capsule 3. Tension lines from instrument

You can therefore see the reflections of the operation lights. They tend to be flitting and are seen along the radiating tension lines that spread out from the point of contact with your instrument towards the periphery. You may occasionally see horizontal folds in the capsule if it is very lax.

Remember that virtually all of your manipulations within the eye are controlled by your vision. You get no sensation of feel, no reassuring pressure from the indented capsule. It is all done by observation.

We are likely to encounter a number of difficulties — some quite frequently, others fortunately less often.

Extraction of the cortex at the twelve o'clock position is always difficult, especially if the cannula is blocked by a capsular tag or flap, when it is trapped between the anterior and posterior layers of capsule (Fig. 7.11) and when the pupil begins to constrict.

The cannula port is easily blocked by capsule.

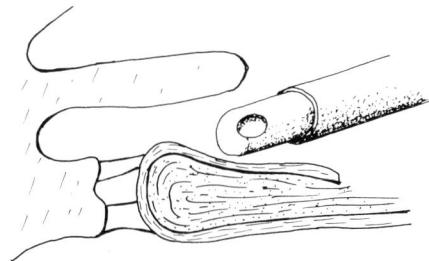

Fig. 7.11 Cortex: Cortex trapped between layers of capsule

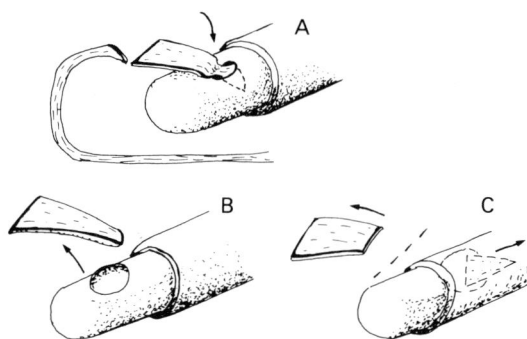

**Fig. 7.12** Cortex: **A** Aspirator blocked by capsule fragment
**B** Capsule regurgitated **C** Capsule abscissed

A small free-floating piece may be ingested or spat
out (Fig. 7.12). If it is attached then you are in
danger of tearing the capsule if you pull on it
(unless it is hanging by a thread). A little pressure
on the syringe will regurgitate the tag, which can
then be dealt with. This is one of the dangers of
fishing under the iris — you are likely to catch a
capsular tag.

You may be able to clear the cannula by using
the double needle as a cutter. Withdraw the
central aspirating needle until the port is covered
by the outer irrigating needle (Fig. 7.12). This
may be difficult to achieve in a controlled manner,
particularly if the needles fit tightly together.

More extensive flaps are best dealt with as
already suggested. A second attempt can then be
made to remove the recalcitrant cortex.

A constricted pupil may tempt you to begin
fishing under the iris and sooner or later you will
catch something that you don't expect and tear the
posterior capsule or produce a zonular dehiscence.
Try iris retraction using a collar-stud retractor
— one of the possible benefits of using the one-
handed syringe; this type of retractor is kinder
than an iris hook. You may be able to elevate the
cornea and proceed with an open sky method
under direct vision. Alternatively do a sector
iridotomy reconstructing a round pupil. I prefer
to do a sector iridectomy as it is the least traumatic
method (Fig. 7.13).

More serious difficulties arise when you tear the
capsule or zonule. These difficulties are
compounded if the vitreous face is also ruptured.
The means of avoiding such problems, or indeed
of dealing with them are considered below.

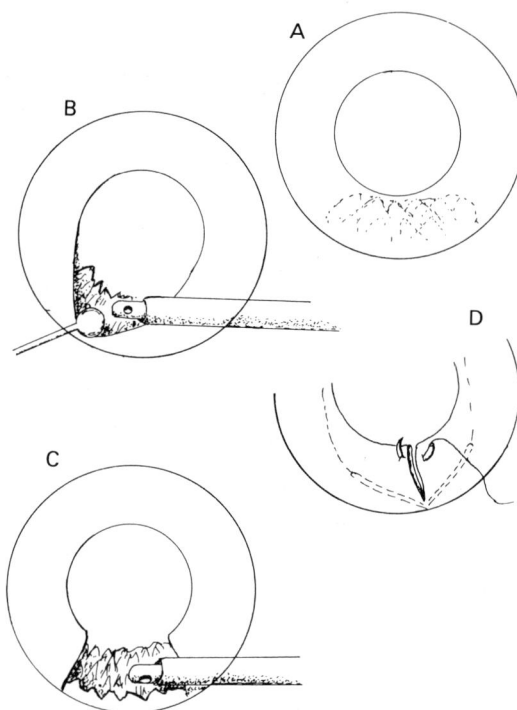

**Fig. 7.13** Cortex: **A** Residual cortex at twelve o'clock **B** Iris
retraction with collar-stud **C** Sector iridectomy **D** Iridotomy
and resuture

Firstly, however, it is important to be able to
recognize a capsular tear or zonular dehiscence
and to know instantly if vitreous is in the anterior
chamber.

## Vitreous

The most unfortunate way to become aware that
you have ruptured the capsule is to observe a
sudden deepening of the anterior chamber
(Fig. 7.14). This happens when the capsule or
zonule are broken and vitreous rushes forwards
into the anterior chamber. In my early days of
extracapsular surgery it soon became my most
frequent cause of vitreous loss — far more so than
with my intracapsular method. This is a disaster.
You have not only lost the many advantages of the
extracapsular approach, but have also compromised your lens implant options and produced a
mess of cortex, capsule and vitreous that will be
difficult to tidy up.

Sometimes you become aware of a vitreous

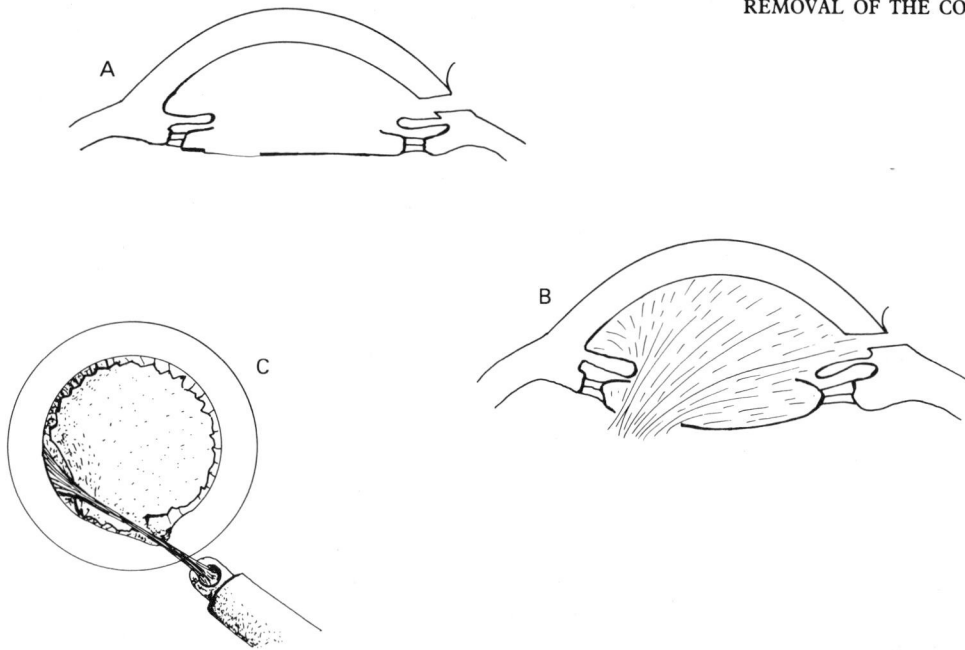

Fig. 7.14 Capsule rupture: **A** Capsule rupture, vitreous face intact **B** AC deepens with ruptured vitreous **C** Vitreous strand

strand on removing an instrument from the eye. It may come through the broken capsule or around the edge of the capsule through an area of ruptured zonule.

Vitreous loss may occur at any time in the procedure but is more likely as the operation procedes. It may occur during the anterior capsulotomy — by tugging on the nucleus or during elevation of the nucleus by zonular stretching — but more commonly it occurs during aspiration and stripping of the cortex and during polishing of the posterior capsule. The causes are the same as those that cause capsule rupture and zonular dehiscence (Fig. 7.15).

The later in the procedure that vitreous loss occurs, the easier it is to manage. If you have already finished extracting the cortex then you must — as for vitreous loss during the intracapsular operation — remove vitreous entirely from the anterior chamber and to the plane of the posterior capsule, by whatever means are at your disposal.

If there is a considerable amount of cortical material left in the eye or if the nucleus is still there then it is more difficult. There is the danger that the nucleus and softer cortical material will sink into the vitreous cavity — never to be

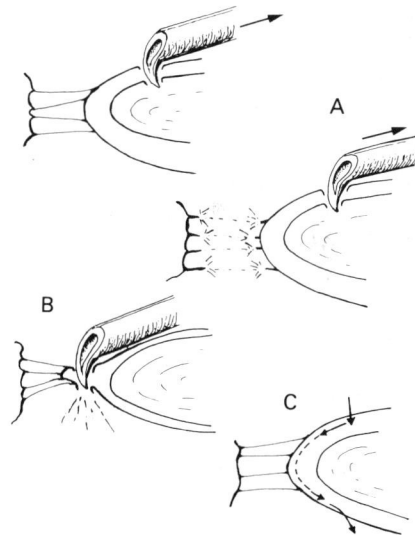

Fig. 7.15 Capsule rupture: **A** Zonule torn during capsulotomy **B** Capsulotomy too peripheral **C** Cutting centrifugally

recovered — to set up a prolonged and severe inflammatory reaction.

You must therefore get the nucleus out first. An old-fashioned vectis, without irrigation, is the best instrument to use. If you attempt to irrigate, bits of cortical material will immediately be dispersed throughout the vitreous. Further expression will of course eject more vitreous and is contraindicated.

Once the nucleus is out or if it has already been removed before the vitreous loss occurs then you must try to remove most of the cortical material. A suction cutter is the easiest instrument with which to remove vitreous, cortex and capsule. If you have only simple instruments then aspiration of liquid vitreous and cortex followed by Weck-Cell sponges for vitreous strands will enable you to retrieve the situation. These procedures involve a lot of extra instrumentation and it is easy with the added excitement of a tense situation to forget about the cornea. Don't. Remember to protect it by lifting it every time you insert an instrument into the anterior chamber and keep the anterior chamber deep so that central corneal touch is avoided. The eye will probably look a mess the following morning unless you keep your head — and are fortunate into the bargain.

Under such circumstances I generally abandon all thoughts of a lens implant. A posterior chamber lens has become impossible, a pupillary fixation lens inadvisable and if really necessary an anterior chamber implant can be done as a secondary procedure, when and if the eye recovers. Do not compound your problems by adding those of a lens implant.

## Capsule rupture

How is a simple rupture of the capsule recognized? I have already discussed at length how to observe the signs by which the structureless capsule is recognized — material on it and reflections coming off it. The absence of these signs indicate an absence of the capsule. So you must constantly be aware of the appearances of the whole posterior capsule (Fig. 7.16). Fortunately there is one postive sign. The area bare of capsule is bounded by bright reflecting lines. These lines are caused by light reflecting and being refracted through the curled up or folded over edges of the torn capsule. The appearance is quite unlike the reflections coming off the surface of the intact capsule. Generally the shape of a capsular tear is triangular, the broader base being towards the periphery.

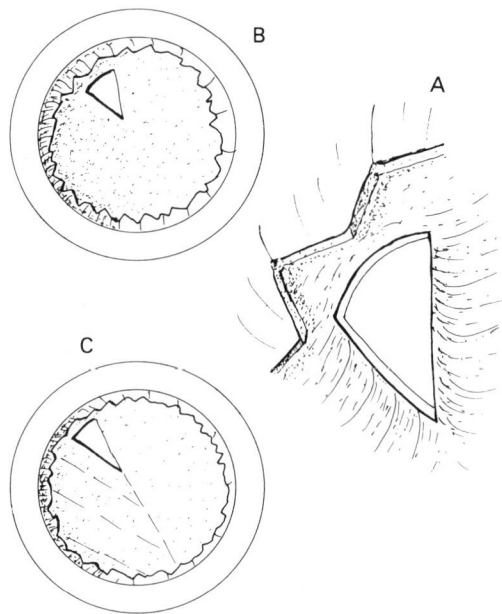

Fig. 7.16 Capsule rupture: A Bright edges of capsule B Small triangular tear C Tears rapidly extend

Tears extend very quickly. As soon as you suspect a tear disengage and withdraw all the instruments from the eye and assess the situation. Confirm that it is a tear, its size, position, the amount and distribution of residual cortical material and the integrity of the vitreous face.

If there is only a little cortical material remaining in the eye it is best to stop further attempts at aspiration. If there is a lot of cortical material still in the eye then you must make an attempt to remove it.

Irrigate and aspirate very slowly and carefully using a low rate of inflow. Keep the tip of the cannula away from the tear and, if stripping, then strip towards the tear. Tension on the capsule is then taken up by that part of the capsule which is still intact and there is little or no pull on the margins of the tear. Any tension transmitted to the capsule surrounding the tear will instantly cause it to extend right across. This is a very difficult manoeuvre to accomplish successfully.

It is a help to tamponade the broken capsule and intact vitreous by using Healon (Fig. 7.17). It may also be possible to uncurl a rolled-up flap of capsule with Healon so that it is repositioned back over the hole. This will help to stabilize the must be looked for (Fig. 7.18). Vitreous may appear from beneath the iris, the implant may disappear or more likely show instability. The only direct sign is an appearance of crescent-shaped lines or folds in the posterior capsule with their concavity towards the periphery, or occasionally the sight of the equator of the capsule with both anterior and posterior layers appearing in the pupil.

Zonular weakness is the main cause of dehiscence. Such weakness is likely to occur with a hypermature cataract, pseudoexfoliation, high myopia and disease such as glaucoma or uveitis.

Factors which may contribute to the dehiscence include pulling the lens too far radially during the capsulotomy, dislocating the nucleus too vigorously, pulling on broad-based capsular flaps during the aspiration, attempting to work through a small pupil and pushing the implant too far down (Fig. 7.19).

So select your patients carefully and perform the anterior capsulotomy correctly — try to remove it all and deal with any flaps. Observation of the capsule through a dilated pupil and clear cornea and the use of coaxial illumination with the eye positioned vertically are vital.

There are certain conditions and manoeuvres that lead to these complications. If you are aware of them and studiously take steps to avoid them then you will reduce the incidence of their occurrence although you will never abolish them completely. We all continue to break capsules at times.

Capsular rupture is more likely to occur if the anterior chamber is shallow or the vitreous/capsule domed and when the pupil is constricted. It may then happen at any stage of the procedure (Figs 7.20 and 7.15).

So once again we come back to those basic needs: keep a soft eye, a deep anterior chamber, the pupil dilated and maintain constant visual control of your aspirator port and polisher with a clear view and appropriate magnification.

The achievement of total cortical removal with the retention of an intact posterior capsule is undoubtedly the hardest part of the whole operation. Time after time you will leave unwanted and often unexpected cortex behind — impossible to remove at the time or only

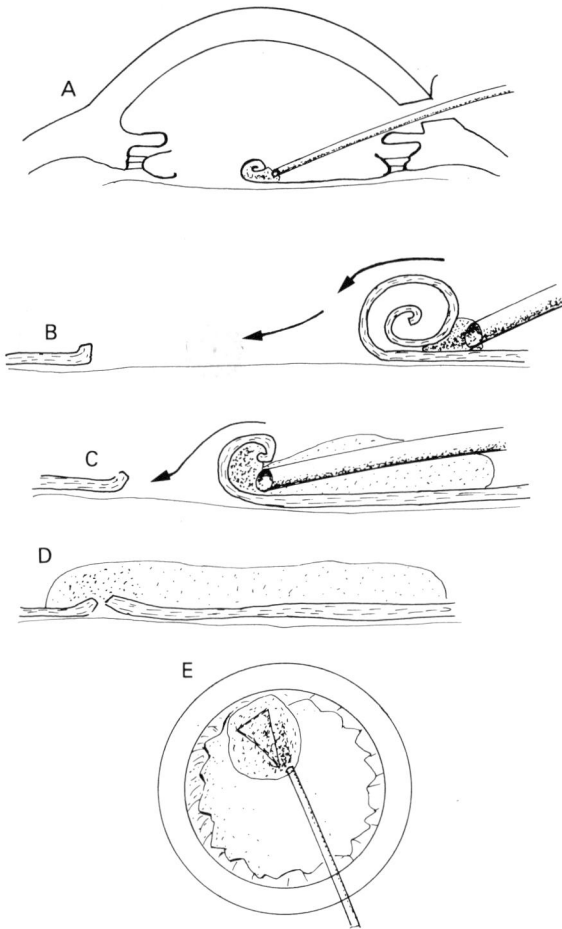

Fig. 7.17 Capsule rupture: **A, B, C, D** Capsule unrolled with Healon **E** Healon tamponade

anterior chamber and protect the vitreous face while you attempt to deal with the remaining cortex. Of course, as you aspirate and irrigate, the Healon will be diluted and removed but it will remain long enough for you to complete an adequate removal of the cortex.

If the capsular tear is small you may proceed to insert your planned implant. If the tear is larger, then a back-up lens will be needed, as I shall discuss in a later chapter.

## Zonular dehiscence

A zonular dehiscence may not be so easy to recognize — even when large — because it is mostly out of sight behind the iris. Indirect signs

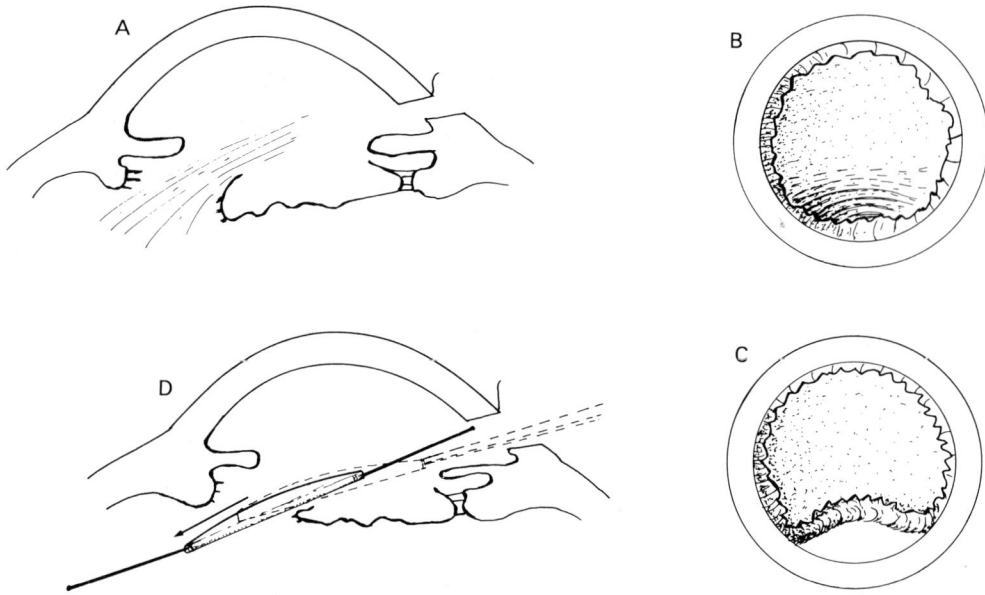

**Fig. 7.18** Zonule rupture: **A** Vitreous in the AC **B** Crescent-shaped lines **C** Equator of capsule **E** Unstable/disappearing implant

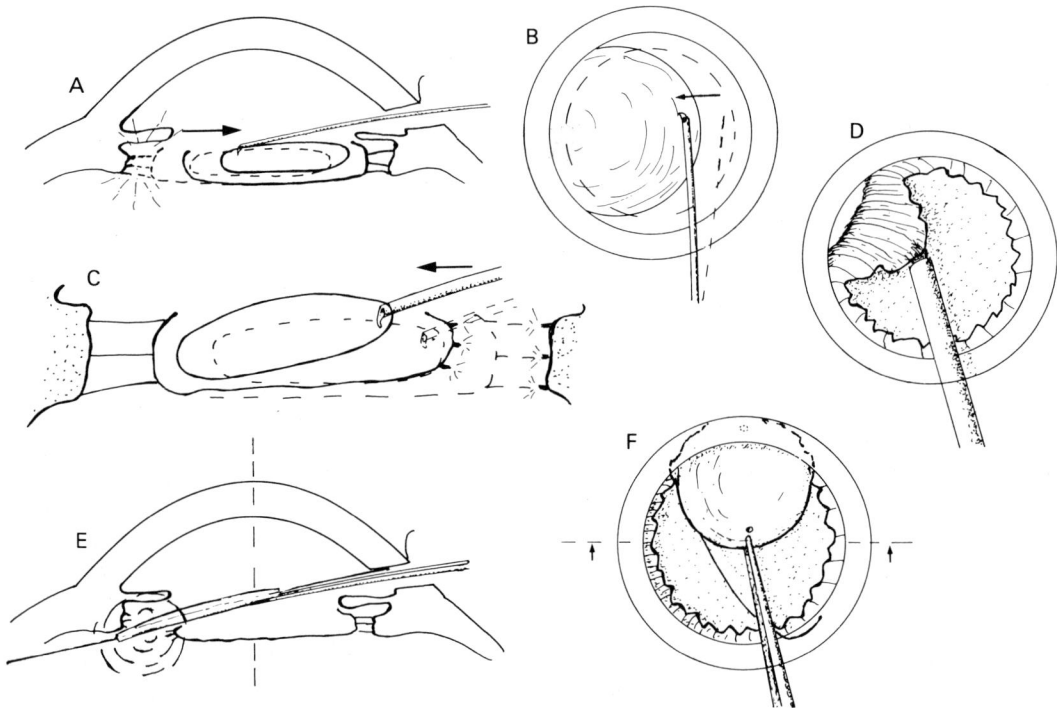

**Fig. 7.19** Zonule rupture: **A, B, C** Pulling nucleus too far **D** Pulling broad-based capsular flap **E, F** Pushing implant below the horizontal

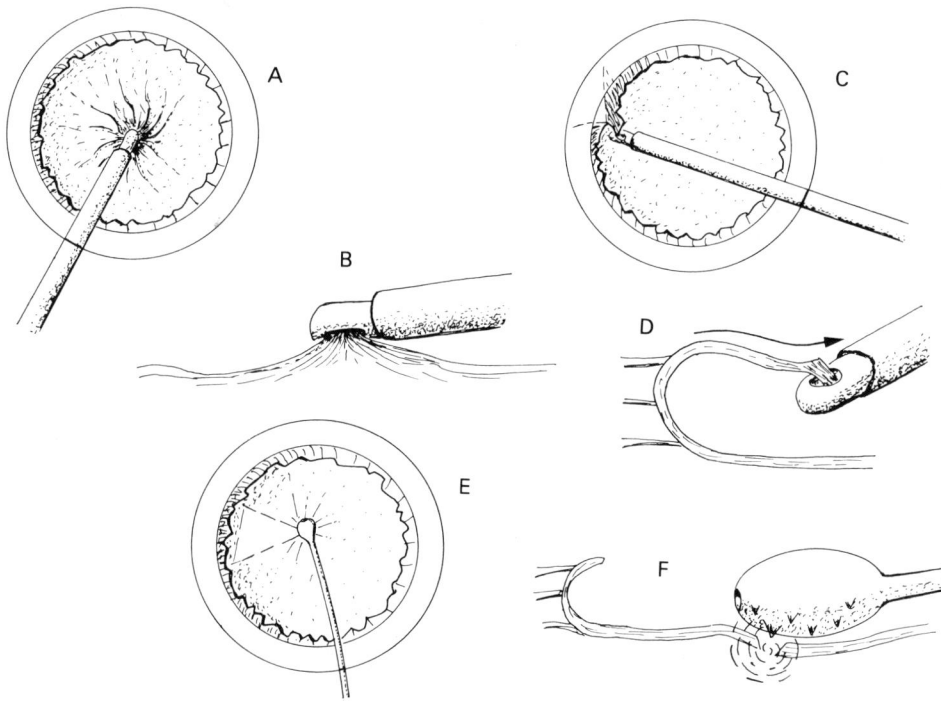

**Fig. 7.20** Capsule rupture: **A, B** Aspiration of capsule **C, D** Pull on capsular flap **E, F** Polishing

revealed while dialling the implant. Sometimes you become aware postoperatively by slit lamp examination or with an extended inflammatory reaction or late tilting of the implant. These are always humbling experiences, particularly when you are beginning to think that you have mastered the technique. There comes an awareness, however, of what is required and what can be done with gradual mastery of the instruments and their characteristics, careful preparation and handling of the eye and the general development of one's observation and by experience. One then enjoys the ability to do an operation quickly, smoothly and without complications so that it is a joy to examine one's patients on the following day's ward round.

This is an exciting and fulfilling task but one which is not necessarily achieved quickly. It may take one or two hundred operations before you are happy with your results and even then you may have had too little experience(!) with the management of complications.

If you have the opportunity and the time you can learn a great deal by watching yourself — action replays on videotape. You may pinpoint obvious errors — why you broke a particular capsule. You may also get a wider view than you are aware of during live surgery, when your concentration is limited to the cannula port or polisher tip. The effect of the instruments on the upper cornea and the actual position of the instruments of expression frequently escape notice, as do the effects of various manoeuvres on the pupil size.

You should now be ready for the implant if this is indicated. The eye is still soft, vitreous and capsule well behind the iris and the anterior chamber deep. The cortex has been cleared away, the pupil is fully dilated and the cornea still clear. Consequently the red reflex is bright. Remember that the retina is sensitive to strong light which is focussed on the fovea once the implant is in the eye. You may get a retinal burn. So protect the macula: turn down the lights or interpose a neutral filter or shield the eye — a blob of Healon or a small swab will do.

# 8

# Modified J-loop
# lens implantation

The essentials:
— insertion in correct place
— preservation of capsule, zonule and cornea
— selection of type and power of lens.
The instruments required:
— McPherson's straight and angled forceps
— Healon
— lens dialler.

There is a huge variety of lenses to bewilder the potential implanter. A recent review of implant types listed no less than 86 modified J-loop lenses alone. There are differences in the manufacturing process, the material of optic or haptic, single or dual material manufacture, the diameter and thickness of the optic and its configuration — biconvex, convex/planar, planar/convex, vaulted or ridged — the overall diameter of the haptics — 11.8 to 14.5 mm — and the number of dialling holes and their size. The loops may be white or blue and of different gauge of thickness and different lengths. The optic may if required incorporate an ultraviolet filter. The haptics may be in line with the optic or variously angled forwards between 7 and 10 degrees. Some lenses are available 'left handed'. The method of sterilization varies. The available powers range from +6.0 to +30.0 dioptres, in steps of 0.5 or 1.0 dioptres. There is also a range of prices.

Each manufacturer tries to offer a similar range of models and will try to stress the importance of any differences in his own range. It is impossible for any surgeon, effectively, to try more than a very few of this formidable list. So the problem is one of selection and choice.

Even subtle and apparently trivial differences in lens design or construction may significantly affect the technique and ease of insertion. I therefore strongly advise the beginner and the surgeon who may not be inserting large numbers of lenses to stick to his selected type until something definitely better comes along. Do not try one or two of this one or half a dozen of that one. It will not help the consistency of your technique or results.

First I shall list what I think are the more important features of these types of lenses and indicate the choice that I have made for my own particular method.

1. *Track record.* I use a well-tried lens style. Most of the difficulties and complications are already known.
2. *Single or dual material.* Single material lenses of PMMA may be safer biologically but tend to be stiff. I use a dual material lens for ease of insertion.
3. *Manufacturer.* Look for a well-established firm with a good reputation. Lathe cut or injection moulding is less important than quality control.
4. *Sterilization.* The dry method is more convenient.
5. *Presentation.* I choose a method which reduces handling of the implant to a minimum.
6. *Price and service.* Discounts are often available and a variety of services offered — replacement or return of non-implanted lenses, special power lenses.
7. *Size.* This is largely determined by the choice of sulcus fixation. I find sulcus fixation easier than attempting to insert in 'the bag', and therefore use lenses of 13.5–14.5 mm.
8. *Laser ridge or posterior concave.* The growing popularity of laser capsulotomy makes a gap between implant and capsule useful.
9. *UV filtration.* These lenses may reduce cystoid macular oedema.
10. *Colour of haptic.* Blue is easier to see.

You seldom obtain all of your requirements in one brand and model. Choose the most important factors and then give that lens a fair trial.

## Lens powers

This subject will be investigated fully in a later chapter. Initially you will be choosing patients known to be emmetropic and therefore probably using a standard power lens of 21.0 D in the posterior chamber, if you have no means of measuring axial lengths. Rules of thumb for correcting ametropia are largely guesswork and even emmetropic patients may have unusual dimensions. So surprises of up to 8 or 9 D of myopia occasionally occur. It is a great disappointment to end up with such a result after a technically successful operation, and little short of a disaster if the patient has good vision in his other and emmetropic eye. If you measure, then the range of powers required will gradually extend and you may find it necessary to use half-dioptre steps as your measurements become increasingly accurate.

## Lens sizes

The correct length for most eyes is 13.5 mm for sulcus fixation, unless the cornea is large. This is usually seen in a myopic eye so it is unlikely that you will be implanting in such cases to start with. If your scope widens to include myopes then you will need a few larger lenses of 14.0 or 14.5 mm diameter in powers of 10 to 15 dioptres.

## Insertion of the lens into the correct place

The ciliary sulcus is an anatomical entity only in the presence of an intact zonule and posterior capsule. The loop of the lens must therefore be correctly positioned in the sulcus between the posterior root of the iris and the ciliary body. Subsequent fibrosis produces permanent fixation of the lens. It is easy to insert correctly provided that it is not caught in a capsular bag or lost through a zonular dehiscence.

## Insertion

In the first instance let us imagine that we have

an ideal patient in whom to insert a lens implant. The cornea is clear, the anterior chamber deep, the iris and posterior capsule in a horizontal plane. The pupil is widely dilated and there is a good red reflex. We are going to use a Sinskey style lens with blue loops angled 10 degrees forwards. These are the steps that will be taken, by a right-handed surgeon.

1. Check the lens for type and power.
2. Take the straight McPherson's forceps in the left hand and the angled McPherson's forceps in the right hand.
3. Pick up the implant by the loop furthest away from you — this will become the inferior loop — with the straight forceps held in your left hand. Hold the loop about half-way along (Fig. 8.1).
4. Irrigate with BSS.
5. Bring the implant into the microscopic field.
6. Grasp the edge of the implant — near the upper dialling hole — with the angled forceps held in your right hand. Make sure you have a firm

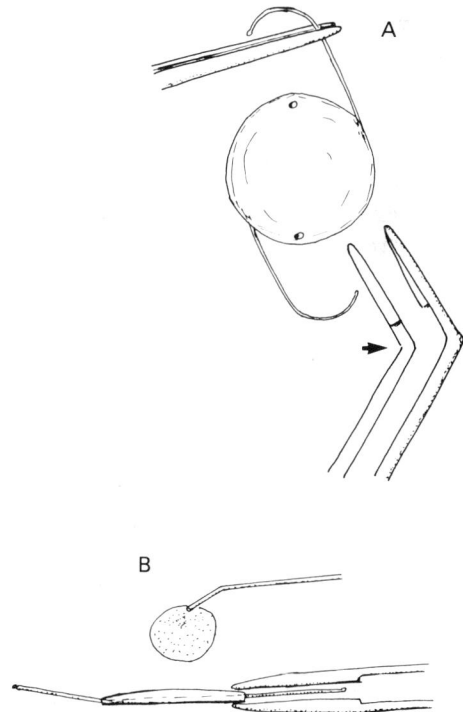

**Fig. 8.1** Implant: **A** Lower loop is grasped half-way along. Position angled forceps with 'elbow' to right **B** Put Healon on the implant

enough grip. Hold it too near the edge and it will flip away like a tiddly-wink. Your hand should be in the prone position with the angle of the forceps directed towards your right.

This sequence of movements is the minimum that will allow you to position the lens correctly for insertion. It avoids unnecessary touching or scratching of the optic during preliminary lifting and positioning. You can then place the right-hand forceps accurately, while you view under the microscope.

7. Inspect the implant to make sure it is the correct way round — convex surface anterior and loops angled forwards.
8. Place a blob of Healon onto the surface of the lens (Fig. 8.1).
9. Lift the edge of the cornea a little with the left hand.
10. Angle the implant 10 degrees downwards so that the inferior loop is in the same plane as the iris (Fig. 8.2).

With the angle or elbow of the forceps to the right your wrist and fingers are in the easiest position to angle the lens the necessary 10 degrees downwards. If you don't do this then the inferior loop will advance anterior to the iris. A further corrective movement will then be needed to readjust it.

11. Slip the lens into the anterior chamber from a position just to the right of twelve o'clock down towards six o'clock. This is easier for the right-handed person.
12. The inferior loop will go beneath the iris at six o'clock.
13. Release your hold on the lens optic as the angled forceps reach the wound edge. Don't push them right into the eye.

There is no need to put the forceps into the eye. If you force the optic into the centre of the pupil it will only spring up again and you risk stretching the zonule. In addition, if the forceps are inside the eye they can only be released by opening the

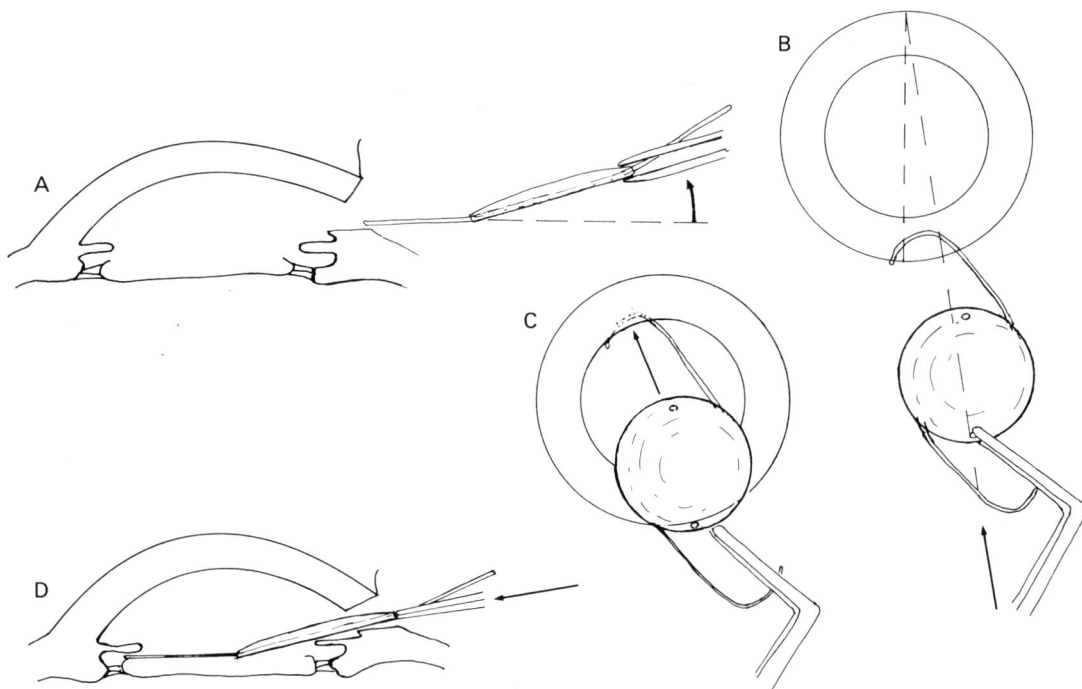

Fig. 8.2 Implant: A Angle implant 10 degrees B Introduce from right of twelve o'clock C, D Nudge opitc into AC with closed forceps

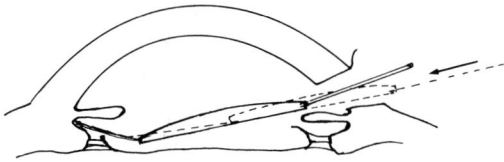

Fig. 8.3 Implant: Nudge optic into AC

tips in an anterior posterior direction — that is towards the cornea. Even if you do not touch the central cornea you will certainly damage the peripheral cornea.

14. Nudge the optic of the lens into the anterior chamber using the closed tips of the angled forceps against the edge of the optic (Fig. 8.3). It is easy to keep the closed forceps in the same plane as the lens optic and nudge it sufficiently into the anterior chamber, thus avoiding possible damage to the cornea.

15. The lens will go over the scleral rim into the anterior chamber — sometimes completely, sometimes partly. Push it in.

16. Take the angled forceps with their angle or elbow directed towards your left and with your right hand in the supine position, then grasp the free end of the upper loop by its tip (Fig. 8.4).

17. Pronate your left hand a little; i.e., roll the palm to your left. This rotates the upper end of the angled forceps to the left, the centre of the rotation being the tip of the upper loop; 20–30 degrees is enough.

These are the key movements for positioning the upper loop successfully. The movement of pronation twists the loop into a backward curve. This backward curve brings the major part of the loop behind the iris as it crosses the pupil margin. The hand positions for these key movements are illustrated in Figs 8.5 and 8.6.

18. Slip the forceps into the anterior chamber and aim towards the edge of the iris at the three o'clock position; that is, half-way down on the right. If you aim towards three o'clock then the loop bends near its junction with the optic so that

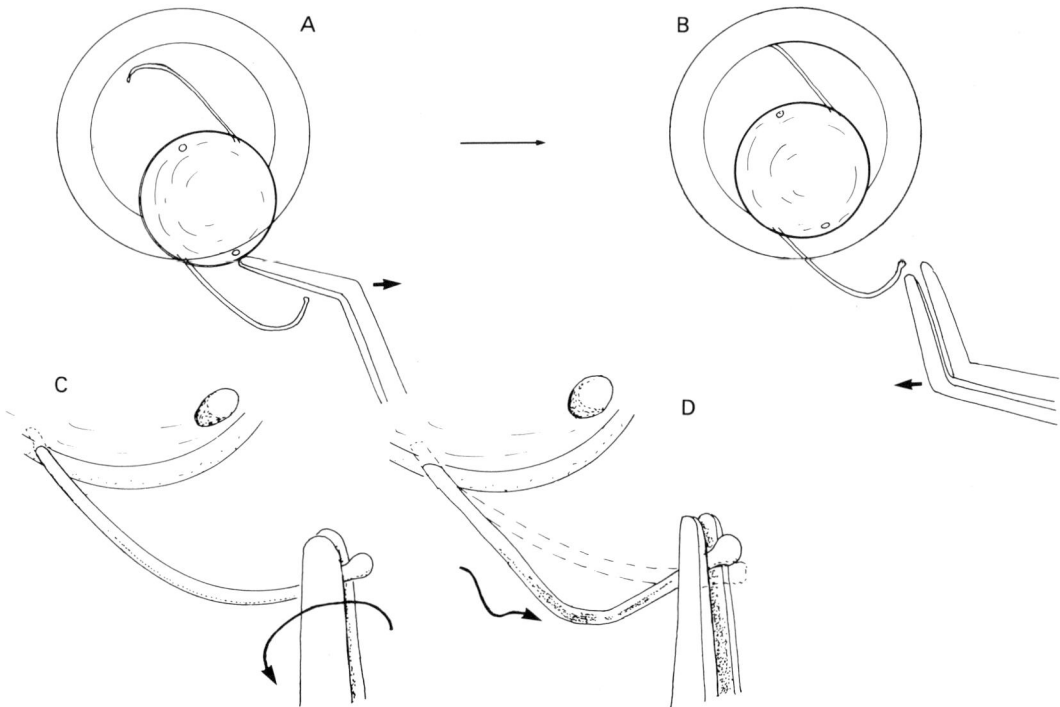

Fig. 8.4 Implant: A, B Rotate angled forceps until 'elbow' points points to left, hand in supination C, D Grasp tip of loop and rotate back, 15–20 degrees, hand in pronation

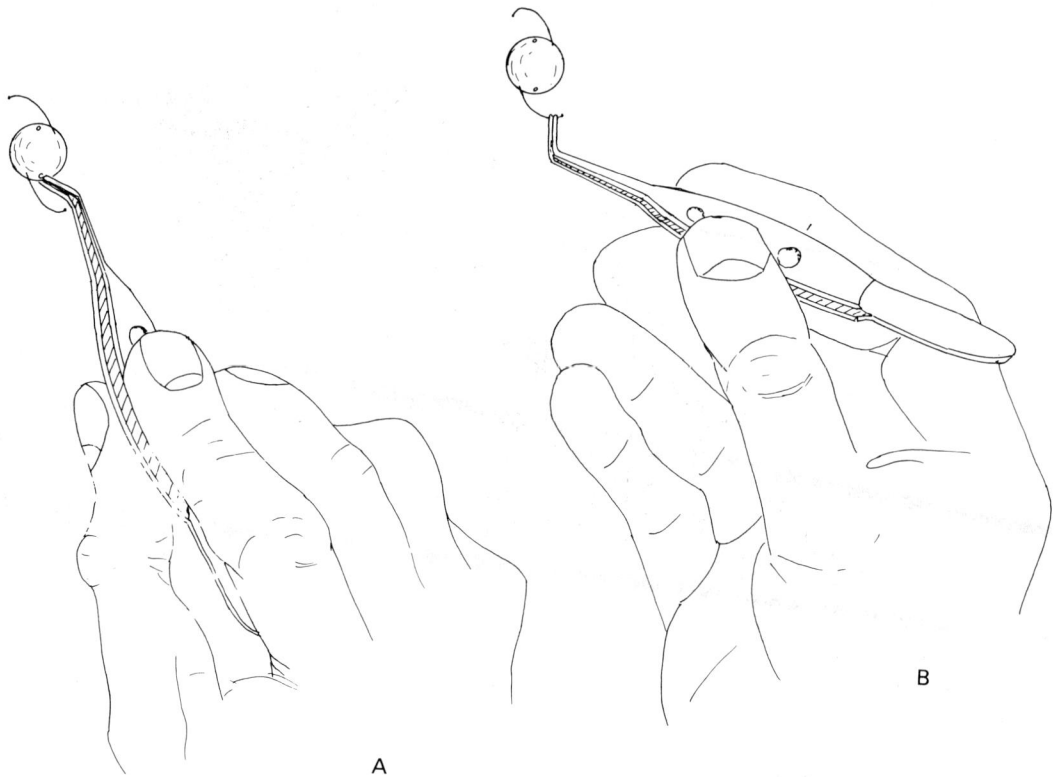

**Fig. 8.5** Implant: **A** Grasp optic with hand in prone position **B** Grasp loop with hand in supine position

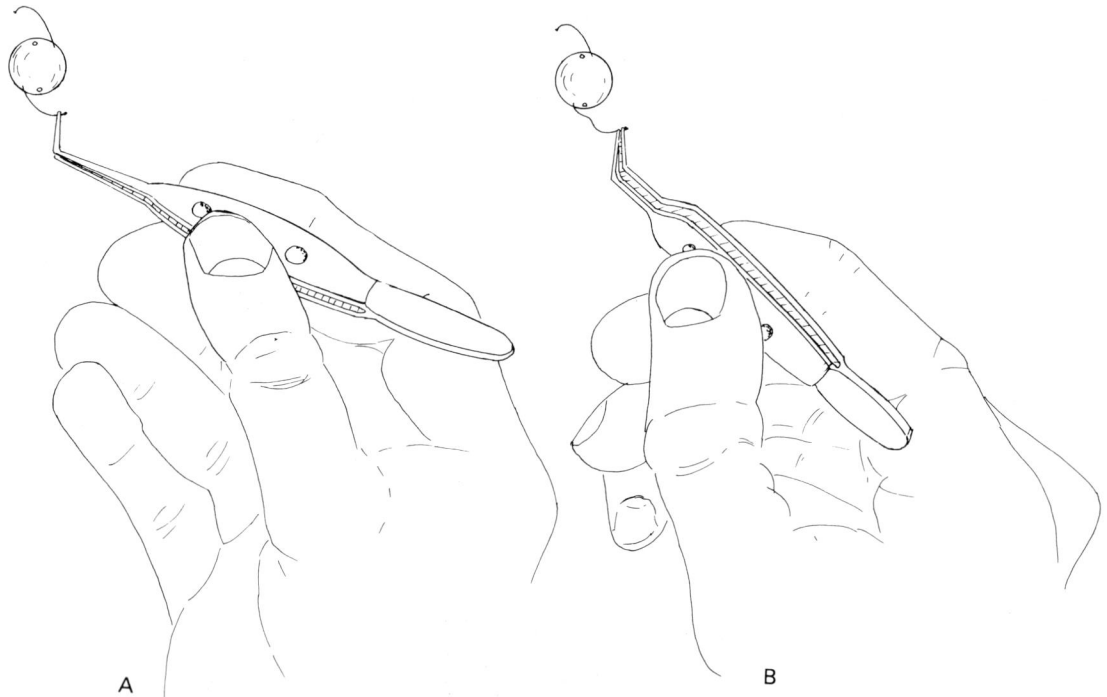

**Fig. 8.6** Implant: **A, B** Pronate hand 10–15 degrees to twist loop

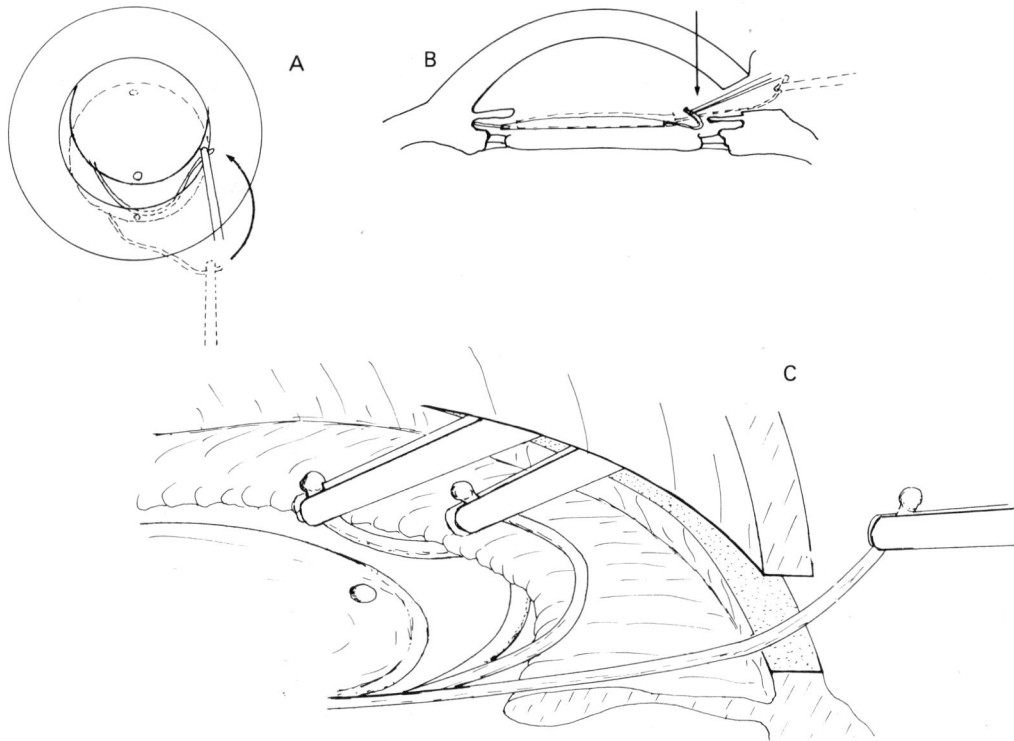

**Fig. 8.7** Implant: **A** Take tip of loop to nine o'clock position **B** Loop crosses pupil margin **C** Movement of loop during insertion

downward displacement of the optic and inferior loop are kept to a minimum.

19. As soon as the bend of the upper loop crosses the iris margin it will take up a position posterior to the iris. Then release the tip of the loop. The loop will spring up behind the iris. Withdraw the forceps from the eye (Fig. 8.7).

20. Do not allow the body of the lens to be pushed below the horizontal. The lens is now wholly in the posterior chamber.

21. Insert the dialler into the anterior chamber. Place its tip into the dialling hole at the top and dial 20–30 degrees. Repeat using the lower hole and again with the upper hole, each time dialling clockwise until the dialling holes are positioned at nine and three o'clock and the two loops are lying in the horizontal (Fig. 8.8).

22. Now nudge the upper edge of the optic in a downwards direction with the the tip of the dialler. It should spring up again immediately, indicating that the zonules are intact. If it does not spring up then either the zonule is deficient or the

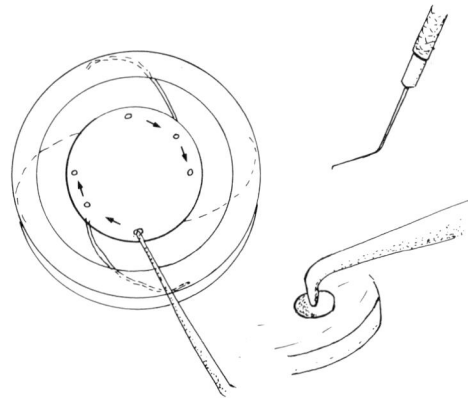

**Fig. 8.8** Implant: Dialling, 20 degrees at a time

implant is too small. Rotate the lens a few more degrees and try again (Fig. 8.9).

Unlike most of the rest of the extracapsular procedure this very important manoeuvre can be well simulated in the practice situation. You should practise this sequence of 20 odd move-

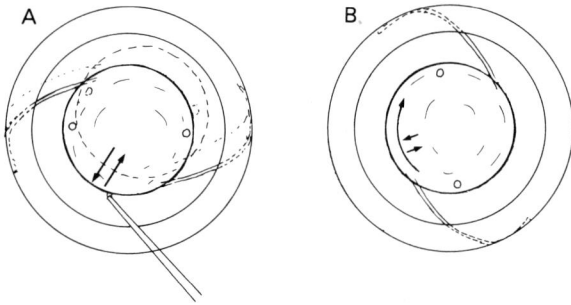

**Fig. 8.9** Implant: **A** Tap test **B** Rotate implant and repeat if unstable

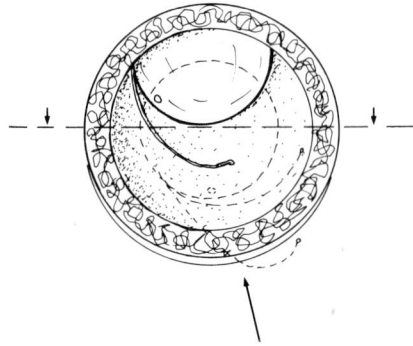

**Fig. 8.11** Implant: Loop directed to twelve o'clock, optic pushed below horizontal

ments on a practice silicone eye, using the actual instruments that you will use, until you have perfected them.

In this ideal situation all difficulties will come from not following this procedure. You will either add extra and unnecessary movements or the lens will not go into the right place. You will therefore inflict unnecessary injury upon the eye and may scratch or deform the implant.

There are several common mistakes. The lens optic and forceps should not be pushed right into the eye (Fig. 8.10) as this will injure the cornea.

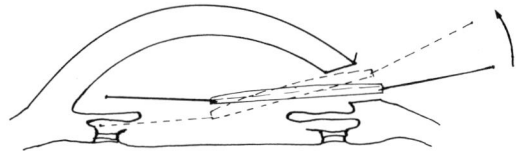

**Fig. 8.12** Implant: Implant not angled enough

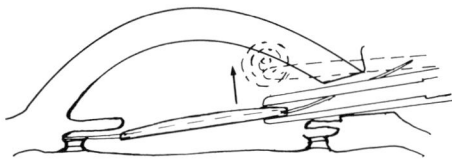

**Fig. 8.10** Implant: Endothelial trauma from opened forceps

The upper loop is grasped other than by its tip. The upper loop is pushed towards twelve o'clock and the lens optic below the horizontal (Fig. 8.11). The lens body is not angled downwards so that the inferior loop lies anterior to the iris (Fig. 8.12).

All these mistakes can be readily readjusted, but why not learn to do them in the least complicated and smoothest fashion from the beginning? It will be quicker and slicker, and can do no harm to your reputation as a surgeon.

For your first attempts at implant insertion you should strive to attain ideal conditions. If you do make one or two minor errors recovery is not too difficult and the eye is unlikely to suffer. Don't become impatient if these ideal conditions seem

to elude you. I recall waiting some two months before putting in my first implant — successfully.

The two problems most likely to cause you to abandon thoughts of an implant are constriction of the pupil and bulging of the iris/capsule/vitreous which produces a shallow anterior chamber. These are of course two of the factors to which so much attention has been paid throughout the whole of the preliminary extracapsular procedure. It is now that the carefully prepared and executed operation reaps further dividends by an easy implant insertion.

If the pupil is constricted to less than 6 mm, which is less than the diameter of the optic, and the anterior chamber is still deep then the optic will not slip directly into the posterior chamber after insertion (Fig. 8.13). Position the inferior loop as before — it is actually easier to put it under the iris when the pupil is small. Release the body of the lens and nudge it as before; the lower rim will lie in the pupil and most of the lens on the surface of the iris. Leave it there. Grasp the tip of the upper loop and manoeuvre it as before. Be sure to push it well down to the three o'clock position. You will have to bend it behind the optic until the loop slips behind the iris. Then release it.

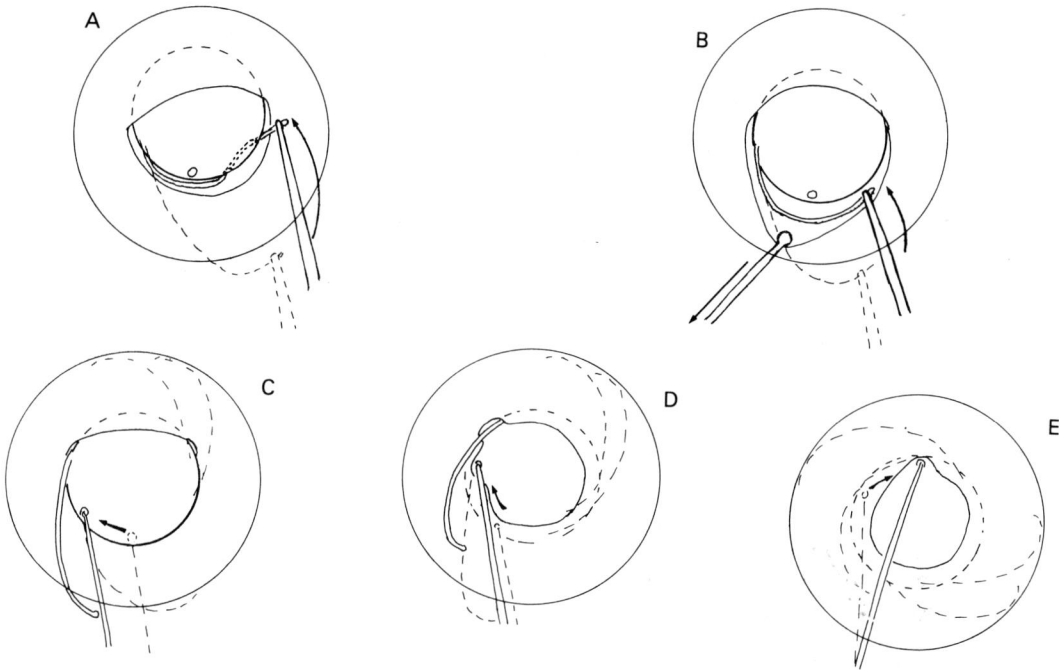

**Fig. 8.13** Implant: **A** Loop bent behind optic **B** Iris retraction, two handed **C, D, E** Dialling it all the way

You now have both loops behind the iris and the optic in the anterior chamber or wedged in the pupil. There is no tendency for the optic to rise or twist towards the cornea. Put in the dialler as before. The lens optic passes easily through the pupil into the posterior chamber as you dial. Dial to the horizontal position.

If you do not like the idea of bending the lens loop so much then you can adopt a two-handed method. Proceed as indicated until you have

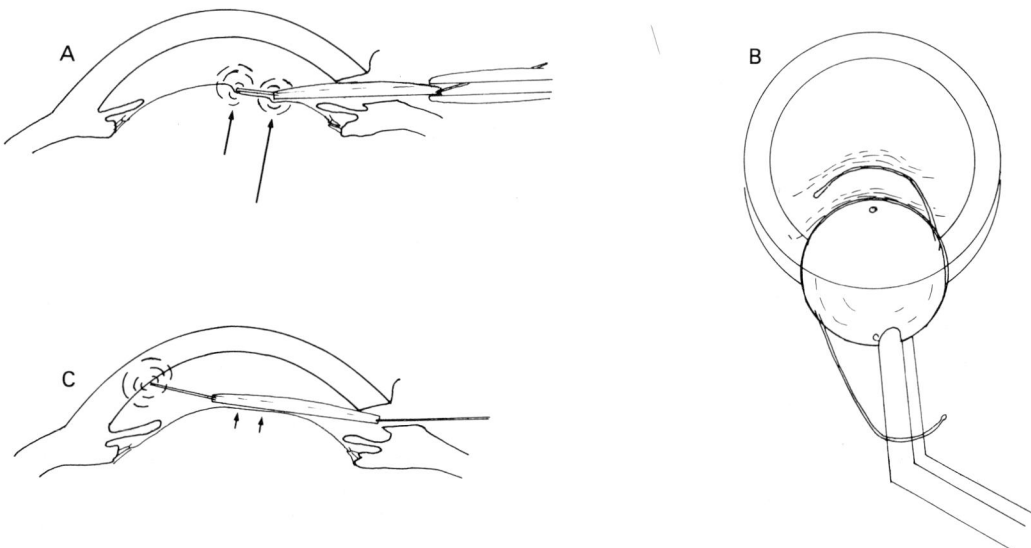

**Fig. 8.14** Implant: **A, B** Loop and optic impinge on capsule/vitreous **C** Loop 'misses' the pupil margin

grasped the tip of the upper loop. Then introduce an iris hook with your left hand. Retract the iris enough to allow your upper loop to slip behind the iris. Dial as before. As a further alternative the lens may be dialled in all the way (Fig. 8.13).

Our second problem arises when the capsule and vitreous start to bulge — perhaps a rebound from the balloon. This situation is slightly harder to manage when the pupil is fully dilated than when partly constricted.

If you now try to insert the lens the inferior loop will impinge upon the domed central capsule and may get stuck and threaten to tear it (Fig. 8.14). Further efforts to introduce it may cause the leading edge of the optic to impinge similarly upon the capsule. You may be able to elevate the loop and body over the domed capsule. You will then find that the inferior loop passes anterior to the iris at the bottom and may rub against the cornea. Any efforts to lift the upper cornea to allow a steeper angle of entry are likely to fail and inflict more corneal injury. There is no way forward.

It is possible to guide the inferior loop to the side of the dome thereby reaching the retro-iris space between three and seven o'clock (Fig. 8.15). You can then slide the optic back to the centre.

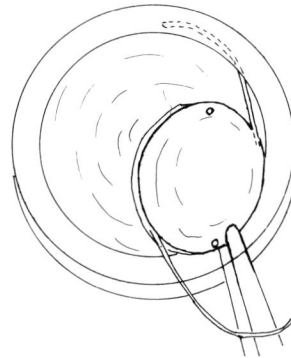

Fig. 8.15 Implant: Implant: Implant slides around the side of domed capsule

This only works with a relatively small dome.

If your initial attempt has failed it is far easier and safer to withdraw the lens and take precautionary action. Inject Healon over the central bulging dome of capsule (Fig. 8.16). You must put it exactly where you want it. Watch the dome being flattened and continue until it is once again in a horizontal plane. Then proceed with your lens insertion, which will now be straight-forward. If difficulty is still experienced inject a small amount of Healon beneath the iris at the six o'clock position. This will lift, 'tent', the edge of

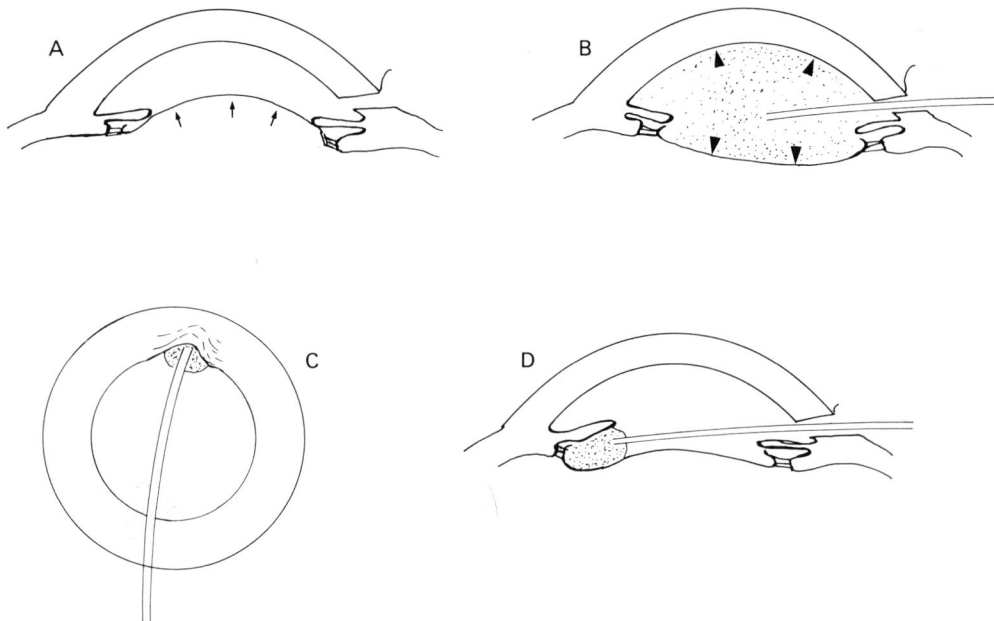

Fig. 8.16 Implant: A Vitreous pressure B AC deepened with Healon C, D Iris 'tented' at six o'clock with Healon

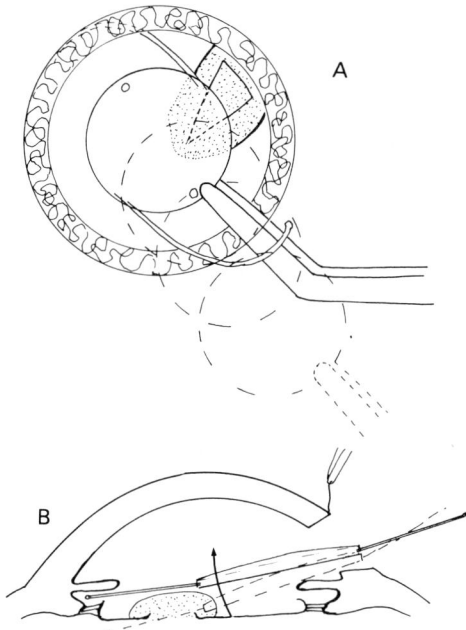

Fig. 8.17 Implant: **A, B** Tamponade tear in capsule and steer implant away from tear

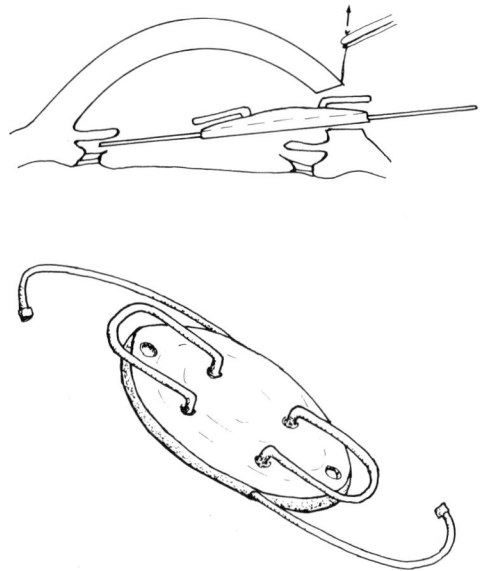

Fig. 8.18 Implant: The Faulkner lens

the pupil and allow the loop to pass easily behind the iris. It is easy to maintain a deep anterior chamber if you use Healon; only rarely will you have to close the incision. Remember that you will have to wash out the Healon at the end of the operation.

## CAPSULAR TEARS, ZONULAR DEHISCENCE AND VITREOUS LOSS

Capsular tears, zonular dehiscence and vitreous loss are more difficult complications to deal with.

### Capsular tears

A small circumscribed capsular tear is not a contraindication to a modified J-loop lens implant. Use Healon to tamponade the tear and proceed with extra caution (Fig. 8.17). Make sure the inferior loop passes anterior to the tear and reduce movement of the lens optic to a minimum. Avoid dialling. This will reduce stretching of the capsule and zonule which will enlarge the tear.

An eye with a large tear or a tear that extends

to the periphery with involvement of the zonule is unlikely to be able to support a lens of this type. You must therefore have a back-up lens available.

I use the Faulkner (Fig. 8.18). This is a modified J-loop with the addition of two anterior loops for pupillary fixation. Tamponade the tear. The lens is inserted in a similar way. It is however a two-plane lens. The cornea must be lifted higher and needs greater protection. The loop must be directed to a peripheral area away from the capsular tear. Once such a position has been achieved do not dial. Pupillary constriction will aid centring and fixation until capsular fixation has occurred. The pupil may then be safely dilated. Remember to do a peripheral iridectomy when using pupillary fixation.

### Zonular dehiscence

Small zonular dehiscences may be quite common. Always test the implant's fixation and, if it does not spring up, rotate it a little more. Greater and visible dehiscences are more troublesome if at the sides or below. Use the back-up lens if less than a quarter of the circumference; if larger then consider a second back-up lens, pupillary or anterior chamber or, if in doubt, wait and at a later date consider a secondary implant. If the dehiscence is confined to the upper region and the zonule is still intact below proceed with the usual implant, but make the initial insertion as oblique as possible.

## Vitreous loss

I think that vitreous loss — except in the rare instance of a very small loss through a limited tear or dehiscence — is a definite reason for abandoning the implant. The few occasions when I have not done so have been unsuccessful. In one patient a 'setting sun' syndrome, which required lens removal followed by an apparently successful anterior chamber insertion and the recovery of 6/12 vision, was finally complicated by a severe cystoid macular oedema and a final reduction of vision to a permanent count fingers. Then there was a case of pupillary block, after a pupillary fixation implant where vitreous came through the pupil. A vitrectomy and iridectomy were successfully carried out through a *pars plana* approach, relieving the block. Permanent peripheral anterior synechiae however produced a severe secondary closed angle and the need for a drainage operation, not an easy procedure in the presence of a pupillary implant. She is lucky to retain 6/18 vision.

It is better to confess your failure to implant and at least let the eye live to fight another day.

# 9

# Postoperative care and complications

The essentials of routine postoperative care are:
— control of uveitis
— control of the pupil
— control of ocular pressure.

The early phase of postoperative care, between the operation and about six to eight weeks — when glasses are prescribed — is dominated by these three problems: the control of uveitis, the control of the pupil and control of the ocular pressure.

## UVEITIS

Let us first consider control of uveitis. I have already mentioned pre-existing uveitis as a contraindication to lens implantation, although the extracapsular approach is often needed in younger persons with cataract caused by uveitis. All patients undergoing extracapsular extraction with or without an implant will develop uveitis, which may vary from the minor and transient to the protracted, severe and recurrent. Steps must therefore be taken to avoid and minimize its worst effects.

Iritis, if not pre-existing, arises from injury to intraocular tissues — particularly the iris, from the effects of release of lens material and from reactions to the materials associated with the implant.

Try to be wise before the event. Be suspicious of the unilateral cataract or the presence of cataract in the younger person. Your preoperative assessment may reveal one or two K.P.s or some decoloration of the iris. During and after the operation you may reduce the production of inflammatory mediators by blocking the ciliary ganglion, by the use of prostaglandin inhibitors

and by relieving pain. You must also keep intraocular manipulation and trauma to a minimum. Try to remove all the cortical material and follow precisely the manufacturer's instructions regarding the preparation of the implant.

It is most important to review your own technique in detail. Simplify it by cutting out all those movements which are not absolutely necessary and include only those that are. Then perform them smoothly and in sequence without gilding the lily. Know what to do, do it, then stop is the ideal that I strive towards.

If a problem is going to occur, and iritis always does, then you must take steps to treat it in advance. Subconjunctival steroid must be given at the conclusion of the operation. I give a combination of soluble Decadron and slowly released Depot Medrone, 20 mg of each. Postoperatively I prescribe topical steroids from three times a day to every two hours if required. If there is the slightest indication or sign that a severe uveitis is about to start then a short course of systemic steroids should be given. Severe uveitis may take a long time to settle and the sequelae may permanently affect the visual outcome.

When I began to change from the intracapsular with implant to the extracapsular method I did not routinely use subconjunctival steroids. The difference due to the extracapsular method was startling. Much more severe uveitic reactions and a more prolonged response were usual. The response was of two types: an exudative, gelatinous or fibrinous response, usually between three and five days after the operation, and a cellular response occurring between five and twenty-one days postoperatively, often accompanied by a hypopyon.

The results of such attacks of uveitis were bound down pupils, posterior synechiae, deposits on the anterior and posterior lens surfaces, deposits on the posterior capsule, probable capsular opacification and occasionally a vitreous response with permanent opacity formation. The patient's discharge from hospital was often delayed as a consequence or readmission was necessary for intensive treatment. Recovery is then slow — just at a time when vision is usually recovering well. This causes disappointment to everyone.

Since then I have always concluded my operation by injecting steroids subconjunctivally and have had no more severe reactions. Part of the improvement in my results is of course due to improvements in technique and greater experience with the extracapsular method. It is quite clear, however, that for whatever reason there is a significantly greater reaction to the extracapsular operation.

It is also necessary to continue with topical steroids for a fairly lengthy period after operation, sometimes as long as six to eight weeks.

This is different from what one anticipates for an intracapsular operation. Ocasionally, despite such treatment, a reaction may continue with recurrent hypopyons and eventually removal of the offending materials — lens cortex and implant — becomes necessary. I have had to do this on only one occasion. An eye which contained a Binkhorst lens following an extracapsular extraction developed recurrent hypopyons. The reaction could be controlled by intensive steroids but as soon as the dosage was reduced the hypopyon recurred. I removed the implant and residual cortex and posterior capsule, using chymotrypsin. The eye settled immediately and gave no further problem. I still do not know whether the eye had reacted against the implant or its own lens material.

Such reactions have been attributed to mechanical trauma from the implant insertion, toxicity of irrigating solutions, residual implant polishing compounds, residual cortical material or to an immune response to many possible antigens. Any reaction may of course be due to a combination of these factors. A delayed reaction and cellular response do suggest an immune mechanism.

As well as lens material there is a variety of potentially sensitizing substances to which the eye is exposed. The antigen can be introduced with the implant — free monomer, manufacturing additives, products used for finishing. The type of sterilization used is important — ethylene oxide compounds for example may be antigenic. There are several past histories of manufacturing disasters but in general there is a steady decline in the incidence of complications attributable to the design and manufacture of the implant.

These make good reasons for choosing a lens type and manufacturer with a long and trouble-free track record. Stick with a successful combination and be wary about changing without having a very sound reason.

## CONTROL OF THE PUPIL

Control of the pupil is not usually a great problem. At the end of the operation I like to have the pupil constricted to a size smaller than the optic of the implant — less than 6 mm. This often occurs during the procedure.

If it does not then I inject acetylcholine into the anterior chamber or, if the pupil is just bordering the edge of the optic, one drop of 2% pilocarpine applied to the cornea will suffice. Frequently the pupil will not constrict over the optic while the anterior chamber is shallow. So deepen the anterior chamber before deciding whether to use a miotic. Constriction of the pupil will prevent the unlikely event of an early pupil trap should the anterior chamber be lost or become shallow postoperatively.

On the following day I dilate the pupil. Homatropine 2% twice or three times daily is quite sufficient to keep the pupil mobile in most patients. I use a stronger mydriatic only if there is a vigorous iritis or if the pupil is rigid or I have done a sector iridectomy. It is better to overdilate than to fail to dilate enough and quickly enough. Once the pupil has stuck to the lens or been filled with exudate it seldom comes completely free. This may not make a great deal of difference but without a peripheral iridectomy you must take the necessary steps to prevent pupillary block from posterior synechiae. Synechiae to capsular flaps

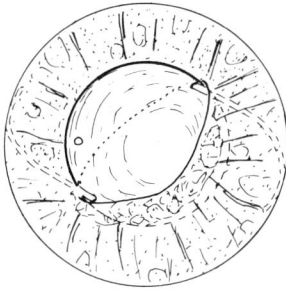

**Fig. 9.1** Pupillary trap

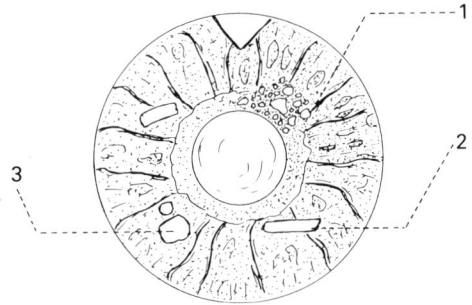

**Fig. 9.2** Iris atrophy: 1. Twelve o'clock position 2. Over the loops 3. From aspirator tip

form more easily than to the surface of the optic. I have seen synechiae form in the dialling holes of the optic, causing fibrosis between the posterior capsule and iris.

Pupillary trap, in which the iris comes to lie between the posterior surface of the implant and posterior capsule, is an occasional complication (Fig. 9.1). It can only occur if the pupil dilates to a size greater than the optic and while in this dilated state the lens optic comes forward or the anterior chamber becomes shallow. Constriction of the pupil then traps the iris behind the optic My impression is that this is more likely to occur if the lens loops are in the same plane as the optic, in which instance the optic lies in a more anterior plane than when the loops are angled 10 degrees forwards. Any period of loss or partial loss of the anterior chamber or the presence of a tear of the iris sphincter — usually produced during removal of the nucleus — may also contribute to pupillary trap, in addition to the aforementioned dilation of the pupil.

Various manoeuvres are described to redilate and reposition the iris anterior to the optic. In my experience they fail unless the entrapment is of very recent origin, as permanent synechiae form very quickly. This is not a complication to worry about unduly. Vision is not greatly affected, although loss of the pupillary reflex may cause glare and the cosmetic appearance is not perfect. Pupillary block glaucoma is unlikely to occur unless the whole of the iris is trapped, itself an uncommon event.

Some degree of iris atrophy is common, particularly in the thin elderly iris (Fig. 9.2). Loss of the pigment layer occurs most frequently during aspiration of the cortex and causes discrete trans-

illumination defects. Widespread atrophy of both pigment and stroma is sometimes seen in the superior iris, as a result of too vigorous manipulation while attempts are made to remove cortex from the difficult twelve o'clock position. Such atrophy sometimes causes obvious pupillary distortion and can be avoided by careful technique. An iridotomy or sector iridectomy will cause less iris damage than over-manipulation and should perhaps be done more often.

## GLAUCOMA

Early postoperative glaucoma, within the first one or two days, is the result of tight sutures or the use of Healon.

Suturing and intraocular pressure have long been a minor problem for the intracapsular surgeon — sometimes made worse by the use of chymotrypsin. Multiple sutures and an absolutely watertight wound — done with the very best of intentions, especially where an iris fixation or anterior chamber lens has been inserted — cause a steep rise in pressure within 48 hours sometimes to above 50 mm Hg. This causes a painful eye and may jeopardize the retinal circulation. A posterior chamber implant following an extracapsular extraction is not accompanied by the same fear of a shallow anterior chamber as in the above conditions. The wound can therefore be sutured accurately and lightly. Such pressure rises are then much less likely.

When Healon has been used during the final phases of the operation — particularly if the anterior chamber has been deepened and the

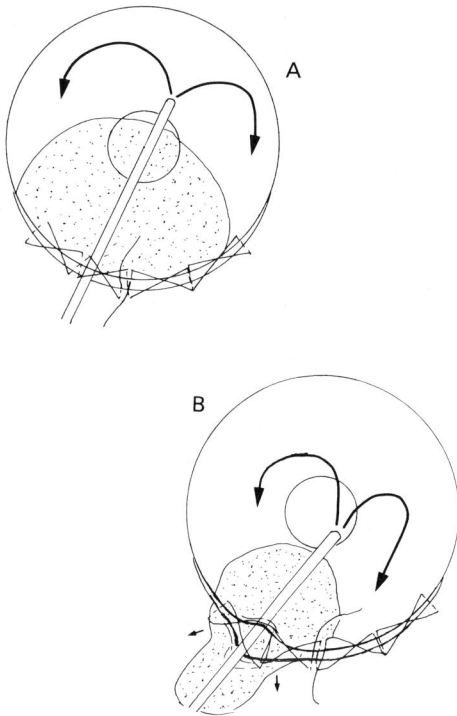

**Fig. 9.3** Glaucoma: **A, B** Removal of Healon

vitreous and capsule repositioned — then the anterior chamber will remain full of Healon for two to three days. This causes a steep rise in pressure, usually late on the following day or night. Pressures of 50 mm Hg with corneal oedema occur. If this does happen then full treatment with diamox and topical timolol must be started immediately. It is preferable to avoid this complication by removing all or most of the Healon at the end of the operation. This can easily be done after suturing of the incision without danger of loss of the anterior chamber (Fig. 9.3). Irrigate the anterior chamber with an air cannula containing balanced salt solution. Pass the tip of the cannula well down into the lower half of the anterior chamber and irrigate. The mass of Healon will be pushed towards the incision above. A little pressure on the posterior lip of the incision will then allow the viscous mass to escape in a rush. Usually it can all be washed out in this way.

If a little remains obdurately in the anterior chamber then just dilute it with balanced salt solution and leave it. You may take precautions,

if more than a little remains behind, by prescribing oral acetazolamide on the evening of the operation or alternatively instilling timolol drops the same evening. It is far better to wash out the Healon at the end of the procedure and allow your patient an uninterrupted night's sleep without extra nursing care.

Glaucoma that develops after three days may be steroid induced or may be open angle glaucoma not known or detected before operation — in the absence of some obvious cause of secondary glaucoma.

The need for use of topical steroid treatment is often prolonged for six to eight weeks. It is therefore not surprising that an occasional steroid reactor appears. It is necessary to measure the intraocular pressure at each postoperative visit. Pressures of 35–40 mm Hg may occur and be a cause of a painful eye and lack of visual recovery. Use of steroids will have to be stopped, curtailed or the preparation will have to be changed according to the need. The pressure will have to be monitored and any hypertension controlled by local timolol or systemic acetazolamide should topical steroids have to be continued. The pressure can be expected to return to normal after a week or two.

Review of such cases has shown a number which had preoperative ocular pressures around the 20/21 mark. Removal of a uniocular cataract on one occasion revealed a cupped optic disc. So beware not only of the well-known uniocular cataract but of the borderline ocular pressure as well. Check it out before operation as far as you can. There is no very great contraindication to performing an extracapsular extraction and implant in a patient with controlled glaucoma. It is sensible however to know beforehand what you may be letting yourself and your patient in for — both in the short term (steroid induced) and in the long term (open angle glaucoma).

## INFECTION

Infection is a rare and disastrous event. The surgeon's suspicions should, therefore, be aroused easily by the warning symptoms and signs.

Any iritis, as we have discussed, should be

looked upon as the beginning of a possible infection.

The pattern may be different from that described for iritis. An onset of symptoms or signs during the first three or four days is significant — the earlier the more significant. Reaction may, however, only occur weeks or even months after the operation. Recurrent attacks of inflammation should also arouse suspicion of possible infection.

A reaction on the first or second day will usually indicate a more virulent organism or perhaps a greater inoculum. A late presentation may indicate a less virulent type of organism, either bacterial or fungal.

The routine use of subconjunctival soluble steroid will suppress the inflammatory response for one to two days, while subconjunctival depot steroids may suppress inflammation for as long as ten days. Subconjunctival antibiotics will modify the response to infection. These modifications may mask the earliest symptoms and signs but will of course buy time for you to make a correct diagnosis and initiate the appropriate treatment.

The first and most important symptom is pain. Never dismiss a postoperative complaint of pain — especially if the immediate postoperative course has been smooth.

Pain is often an indicator of trouble before there are any visible signs on the slit lamp, yet twelve to twenty-four hours later the signs may be only too embarrassingly obvious. It may be that the patient and ward sister have already made arrangements for discharge from the ward that morning. A delay of another day may not be popular but will certainly be justified if severe iritis or infection are thereby detected and treated at an early stage.

Loss of vision is also an early symptom and parallels the degree of reaction and visible signs. The signs are exudate and cells in the anterior chamber and on the implant surfaces initially. Spread through the barrier of the posterior capsule into the anterior vitreous soon follows. This is accompanied by hypopyon, occlusion of a constricted pupil by exudate, and oedema and haziness of the cornea. Visual loss will now be profound.

The early symptoms and signs may be indistinguishable from those of a sterile uveitis.

Diagnosis is obvious if the reaction is overwhelming. It may be strongly suspected if it occurs during the period of maximum steroid suppression or if it is recurrent. Often, however, the diagnosis is in doubt. In these circumstances you must assume the worst and act accordingly, as a delay of one or two days may ensure that vision, if not the eye, is permanently lost. Even with the most favourable result there is only a fifty-fifty chance of saving useful sight.

Once you have decided that action must be taken alert the bacteriologist. A personal contact to acquaint him with the urgent nature of the problem — the likely loss of sight — and the type of inflammatory response is always valuable. You can discuss the specimens that will be available for examination — their nature, amount, method of transportation and culture media. If the specimens are to be collected out of normal hours then arrange for personal delivery of the specimens to a named technician or bacteriologist. It is most important that these vital specimens are not lost and arrive in a fresh condition.

Conjunctival swabs, scrapes or smears are of little value. The best chance of making a diagnosis comes from examination of specimens taken from the aqueous and vitreous.

The bacteriologist may give you assistance — on the basis of the clinical picture — as to the most likely organism and best antibiotic combination to use as a first line attack and will of course give further information when organisms are identified, as occurs in three-quarters of such instances.

The specimens should be collected from the patient under a general anaesthetic. Aspirate from the aqueous using a 25 gauge needle attached to a tuberculin syringe. Penetrate the anterior chamber near the limbus and aspirate 0.1–0.2 ml. Inoculate direct into the medium. The vitreous aspiration is made with a larger bore needle, 22 gauge, through a posterior sclerotomy 4–5 mm from the limbus. Collect 0.2–0.3 ml and transport in a similar way. The specimens are so small in volume that it is worthwhile transporting the needles and tuberculin syringes so that the bacteriologist can make the most of them.

Treatment should begin with immediate systemic antibiotics, preferably intravenous, in maximum dosage to cover the spectrum of likely organisms. Subconjunctival and intracameral antibiotics are given after collecting the specimens. Gentamycin 0.1 mg, cephaloridine 0.25 mg or cefazolin 2.25 mg and amphotericin B 0.005 mg can all be injected into the eye.

The amount of antibiotic that can be injected into the eye without undue toxicity is extremely small. The appropriate dilution should be made up by the surgeon in the operating theatre.

Antibiotics should continue to be administered by all routes until the infection is controlled.

There is a good chance of overcoming or controlling the infection but often only at the expense of intraocular structure and visual function. Steroids should therefore continue to be given throughout the period of treatment so that fibrosis, scarring and toxic damage are reduced to a minimum.

In many instances there is permanent clouding of the vitreous, and vitrectomy at a later stage may clear away the debris and offer some chance of visual recovery.

When the initial inflammatory reaction is severe a vitreous abscess may form. Vitrectomy at an early stage is then indicated. This follows the general surgical principle of draining accumulations of pus and at the same time provides a more generous sample for bacteriological examination.

Finally, there is the question of what to do with the implant. If we again follow the general surgical principle then a foreign body in the presence of inflammation and infection should be removed. Removal of an intraocular lens, especially from the posterior chamber, is difficult enough at the best of times. Attempted removal at such a time and under such circumstances is likely to be so traumatic as to lead to almost certain loss of the eye. It is therefore better to attempt to overcome the infection while leaving the implant in the eye.

Routine postoperative care usually ceases once local treatment has ended and a final refraction has been done. Other complications will be discussed in later chapters.

# 10

# Capsular opacification, secondary capsulotomy, displacement of the implant and retinal detachment

The essentials:
— maintain adequate vision
— avoid unnecessary operations
— keep complications to the minimum.
The instruments required:
— discission knife or needle
— YAG laser.

I have already discussed the indications for the extracapsular method and it is now relevant to discuss in detail the advantages and disadvantages of an intact posterior capsule and those factors which may promote capsular opacification. I shall then describe how to do a secondary posterior capsulotomy. I shall also discuss displacement and instability of the implant and retinal detachment — relatively rare complications.

Throughout this Guide I have tried to promote the search for perfection. I believe this is the goal we should all aim for, not only for the great personal satisfaction that comes from achieving one's very best but for the even greater reward of a patient happily restored to the visual world. This initial restoration may be interrupted by opacification of the posterior capsule, and the need for a second operation. If every operation were done as I have described throughout this Guide and postoperative care was perfect then the need for a secondary capsulotomy would indeed be reduced almost to zero. This is seldom the case and between 5 and 50% of patients required a second operation.

## An intact posterior capsule

The advantages of an intact posterior capsule come from the anatomical and functional barrier that it creates between the anterior and posterior chambers — so-called compartmentalization. This barrier is lost not only when the whole capsule is removed as in an intracapsular extraction but also when the smallest opening or defect is created. There is a greater risk of developing cystoid macular oedema and detachment of the retina when capsular integrity is lost. The intact capsule also offers an increased resistance to the spread of infection.

Most capsules, especially if properly cleaned, allow good vision and will remain clear for life. Routine primary capsulotomy is therefore unnecessary in most patients.

If you intend to do primary capsulotomies on all your patients why bother to do an extracapsular extraction at all? Do an intracapsular and use an anterior chamber lens. It is a lot easier!

There are instances where good vision is unlikely to be regained; for example when there is an obvious capsular plaque or opacity. If it is likely that a secondary capsulotomy will be necessary within the first eight weeks after operation then it is reasonable and better to do it at the time of the first operation. You will have to accept, however, the occasional problem with vitreous strands, cystoid macular oedema and retinal detachment.

I do not do primary capsulotomies — unless I have to. I would also advise you not to do a primary capsulotomy, even where indicated for visual reasons, when there is an increased risk of cystoid macular oedema. A previous episode in the other eye, diabetes or hypertension are such factors.

There is an increased risk of retinal detachment in high myopia and where detachment has occurred in the fellow eye. Primary capsulotomy should therefore be avoided.

A secondary procedure, such as a corneal graft or drainage operation, is also a contraindication to primary capsulotomy, if it is likely to be necessary within a few months.

## Capsular opacification

Most secondary capsulotomies are needed between twelve and twenty-four months after the operation. The need continues, however, for up to four years. It is likely that the longer the interval between the original operation and the secondary capsulotomy the fewer the complications. Therefore wait as long as is reasonably possible.

There is also the ever present danger of endophthalmitis. This is a rare event but may occur after any open operation on the eye with disastrous consequences. This is a strong argument for not attempting secondary capsulotomies other than with a closed method — such as the YAG laser.

The capsule may already be opaque at the time of primary surgery, most often when the cataract is a mature white one. Fibrosis on the capsule occurs when exudative or cellular tissue is deposited thereon. It will therefore follow an attack of uveitis — when fibrinous exudate, white or red blood cells collect. If these tissues are not cleared rapidly they will organize and fibrose. It is doubtful whether the capsule itself undergoes fibrosis.

Residual lens material may also excite a fibrotic reaction. Such reactions will be accelerated if the iris is in direct contact with the capsule.

These factors must be avoided as far as possible by an atraumatic operation and adequate postoperative treatment.

One severe attack of uveitis may be enough to opacify the capsule. Opacification also occurs through attempted regeneration by lens cells and by migration of cells from the iris.

Regeneration from remnants of the epithelium of the anterior capsule will occur if the anterior capsule has not been completely removed. Regeneration also occurs from the epithelial cells in the fornices of the capsular bag, and from lens fibres left behind on the central posterior capsule.

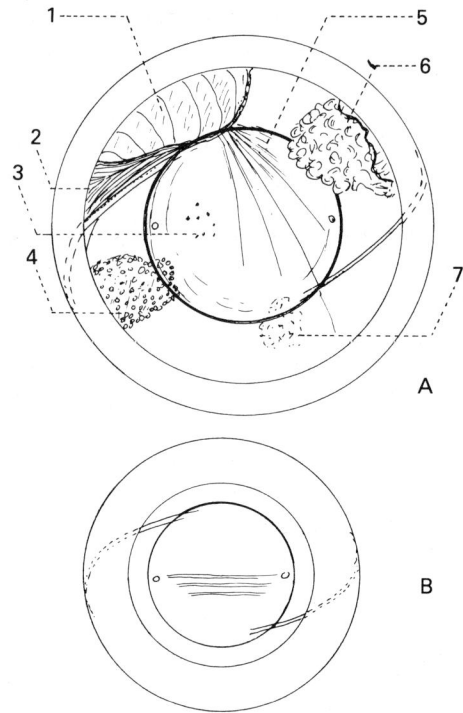

Fig. 10.1 Capsular opacity: **A** 1. Double layer of capsule 2. Dense fibrotic band 3. Deposits on implant surfaces 4. New fibres, 'bubbles', on capsule 5. Tension lines 6. Elschnig's pearls 7. Deposits on posterior capsule **B** Transverse folds in capsule

Regeneration in any of these sites is more active in younger people. Cells from the anterior capsule grow forward to form the characteristic Elschnig's pearls (Fig. 10.1). The visual axis may however remain clear for a long time. Epithelial cells in the capsular fornix grow across the posterior capsule and together with regenerating fibres on the posterior capsule give a bubble-like appearance, most easily seen by retroillumination. This has a marked effect on the visual acuity and is not always effectively treated by simple posterior capsulotomy, as further overgrowth may occlude the opening. Formal capsulectomy may then be necessary.

Capsular folds and adhesions occur after the empty capsular bag collapses. Any residual anterior flap then adheres to the posterior capsule or implant. This is more likely when the posterior capsule is lax or cannot be stretched. It is possible to stretch the posterior capsule and possibly prevent migration of the epithelial cells if a mechanical barrier intervenes — a lens optic of suitable design.

It is often difficult, in the early stages, to know whether a reduction in vision has been caused by capsular opacification — the old problem of macula versus media.

The usual story is of a successful operation with restoration of vision to 6/6. This is followed, nine to twelve months later, by a slight drop in vision over two to three months to 6/9 and 6/12. At this stage there may still be a good view through the capsule and therefore doubts about the function of the macula.

The patient may complain of a variety of symptoms — glare, dazzle, haze, blur and, if you wait long enough, progressive loss of vision. You are then left in no doubt that the capsule is opaque or covered by a membrane. This diagnosis is proved to be correct when vision is restored to 6/6 or sometimes to 6/5, one line better than before, by a capsulotomy. Greater experience aids the recognition of the subtle capsular changes associated with early opacification. Intervention at an earlier stage is therefore sensible. I personally wait until the visual acuity has dropped at least two lines on the Snellen's chart unless the patient is particularly disturbed or handicapped.

Once you have decided that a secondary capsulotomy is necessary then dilate the pupil and examine carefully on the slit lamp. Draw a detailed diagram to show the areas of opacity, their thickness, and the situation of any pearls or stress lines and their relationship to the implant and iris. It is then possible to plan exactly where to make the incision into the eye and where to open the capsule. It is easiest to open thin capsule. Make use of tension lines to widen the opening. A linear opening will then widen sufficiently to make a good gap.

If there is no implant in the eye then an approach through the anterior chamber and pupil is indicated (Fig. 10.2). If there is a lens in the eye then your approach will have to be modified according to the type of lens and the presence or absence of an iridectomy. Introduction of the instrument through an iridectomy is a convenient way of reaching the postimplant space but may not be ideal for your planned manoeuvre. If the

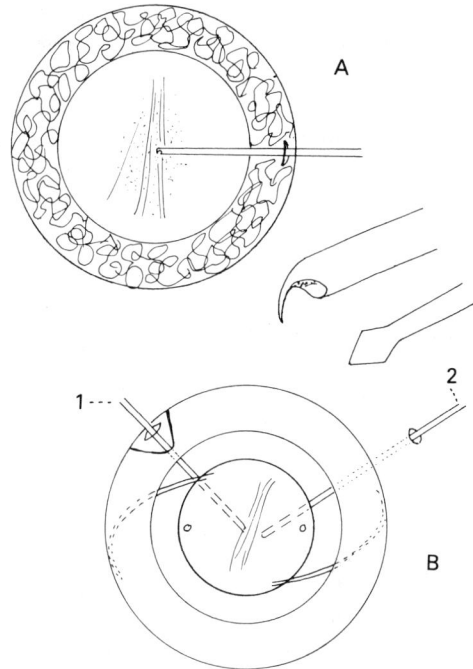

Fig. 10.2 Posterior capsulotomy: **A** Through the cornea **B** 1. Through the iridectomy 2. Through the *pars plana*

pupil dilates well then an anterior approach is possible. If neither of these methods appears feasible then an approach through the *pars plana* can be made.

The view through the slit lamp is always better than that through the operation microscope.

If the pupil does not dilate more than 6 mm, the helpful red reflex which transilluminates the posterior capsule is not obtained. There is then greater difficulty in seeing what has to be done. With good observation it is easy to make an accurate opening, often without rupturing the vitreous face. If observation is poor then rely on the carefully drawn diagram to aid positioning of the needle.

It is easier to manage a capsular fold or thickening than regeneration over the posterior capsule or pearl formation. Anterior groups of pearls may interfere little with vision — so leave them as long as possible. If they must be removed then they should be excised. Attempts at aspiration or efforts to loosen them by polishing or scraping are usually ineffective. Indeed such efforts may only spread the regenerating cells over a wider area.

Cellular spread across the central capsule quickly depresses vision and is difficult to clear. A simple hole made through the capsule remains open only for a short time. The cells continue to regenerate and re-cover the gap. A second attempt at needling is likely to be less successful than the first. If there is no implant present then it is worth polishing or aspirating and stripping the capsule. This does not work very well as the new cells, unfortunately, seem to be very sticky. It is almost impossible to scrape them off or to get a good clear area of capsule. It is better to attempt a wider capsulectomy if the first simpler procedure fails, or to use the laser.

The capsulotomy may be done as an outpatient procedure using the slit lamp and local anaesthesia. I prefer an inpatient procedure, where general anaesthesia and the operation microscope are available. The two requirements are good observation and an appropriate needle.

Observation is achieved with a clear cornea, axially directed eye and lighting, dilated pupil and appropriate magnification.

A Pearce disposable knife or disposable needle with the point bent over the opening are required. A simple stab opening is made and the knife is directed to the chosen spot. The opening in the capsule is then made.

Not many of us have access to a YAG laser. It does the job without opening the eye surgically. There is therefore a reduced incidence of postoperative endophthalmitis, a rare but serious complication. The procedure is under precise optical control — far more accurate than can be achieved manually. There is also no need for the patient to be admitted to hospital.

There are complications — damage to the implant, loss of corneal endothelial cells as well as postoperative uveitis and glucoma. Thin membranes are disrupted easily with very low energy output and complications are minimal. Thick fibrotic membranes, remnants of lens material and regenerating lens fibres require higher energy output. There would however be little or no indication for primary capsulotomy should a YAG laser be available and secondary capsulotomies could more safely be done as simple outpatient procedures.

## Lens displacement

The implant may occasionally become unstable or may truly dislocate. It is then necessary to consider methods for its removal or stabilization.

The 'setting sun' syndrome describes the appearance of the lens implant as it dislocates downwards across the pupil (Fig. 10.3). Initially the upper edge is just visible inside the upper margin of the pupil. As the displacement increases so the lens optic sinks downwards until eventually it disappears as it 'sets' into the vitreous.

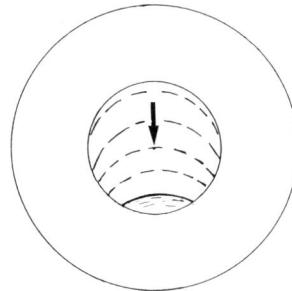

Fig. 10.3 Implant: 'Setting sun' syndrome

The patient may complain of symptoms such as changing focus or double images. There may be an unexpected change in the refraction — increasing myopia or changing and increasing astigmatism — before it becomes obvious that the cause is displacement of the lens. In case of doubt keratometry will determine between corneal and implant induced astigmatism. These events may occur within a few days of the operation but more often they occur several weeks or a month or two after the operation.

These events can only occur if the capsule or zonule is no longer intact. It is usually not difficult to be sure that the capsule is intact, unless the lens insertion was done under very poor conditions — with a small pupil. It is sometimes less easy to be sure about zonular integrity as the zonule is out of sight.

The conditions under which the zonule may rupture have already been stressed. These conditions include: pre-existing weakness as in mature cataract, pseudoexfoliation, myopia, trauma and glaucoma; extra stress from pulling on capsular tags or flaps during aspiration of the cortex; pushing the implant too far down during its insertion. I have also stressed the importance of not pushing the implant below the horizontal and the need for the 'tap' test to ensure that the lens loops are resting in an area where the zonules are intact. If the tap test reveals an unstable lens then it must be rotated further until a stable position is attained.

A lens that dislocates in the first few post-operative days often indicates a large defect in the capsule or zonule. The implant may have disappeared within a few days. Displacement that occurs weeks later is often much slower and it is then a race between displacement and fibrosis. Fibrosis may induce sufficient stability for the implant to remain in a functional if not ideal position. Even when the upper edge of the optic is almost across the centre of the pupil good vision is still possible.

Examination with the slit lamp may reveal vitreous in front of the implant or the torn edge of the capsule or the edge of the capsule where the zonule has come away.

If the implant is obviously dislocating rapidly then you will have to decide whether to remove it immediately, stabilize it or let it fall into the vitreous where it will remain forever. If the displacement is gradual then it is possible to watch for a few days or weeks in the hope that the implant will stabilize while good vision is maintained.

Removal of an implant from the posterior chamber is not easy. No one has much experience with the procedure. The eye is vascular and in an unusually reactive state. Vitreous disturbance, uveitis and cystoid macular oedema are likely as is corneal injury. A successful outcome is problematical even where use is made of viscosurgical aids and where luck is with you.

Begin by dilating the pupil fully and observe the position of the implant's loops. Fill the anterior chamber with Healon through a small stab incision in the cornea (Fig. 10.4). Make another small incision at the opposite side — it is easier to do this before opening the eye. Enlarge the first incision to 7 mm — large enough to remove a 6 mm implant. Introduce a collar-stud retractor or rigid lens dialling hook. Place the tip of the retractor beneath the lens loop where the loop joins the optic. Rotate and elevate the retractor so that the loop comes into the anterior chamber. Grasp the end of the loop with forceps. The situation is now under control. Don't attempt to pull

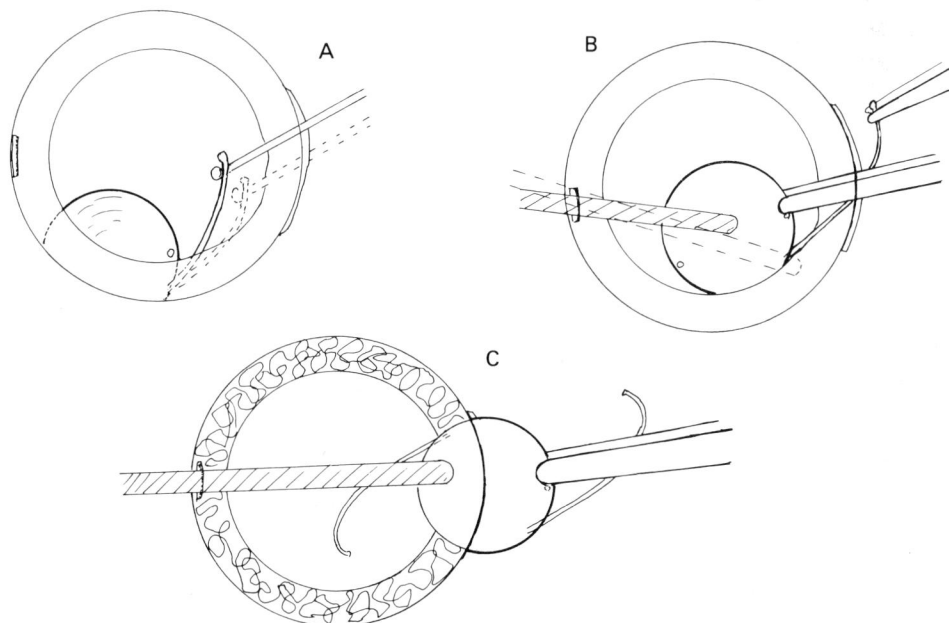

**Fig. 10.4** Implant removal: **A** Retrieve one loop **B** Grasp optic **C** Corneal protection

the implant right out by the loop. The optic will catch on the pupil margin and prevent its removal. The optic will also rotate and touch the corneal endothelium. If there is any difficulty experienced in levering the loop forwards or if the lens optic rotates then introduce a second instrument through the other stab incision and use it as a stabilizer until the upper loop is firmly grasped in the forceps. Now introduce a second pair of plain blocked forceps and grasp the optic by its edge. It can be drawn out through the incision without difficulty.

If one or both loops are fixed and a stable lens has to be removed then a different set of circumstances exists. The optic alone is then removed after cutting through the fixed loops.

I would advise against inserting another implant, even if it is successfully removed, in view of the complications listed above. Should the eye settle satisfactorily and the patient wish it a secondary implant can always be attempted.

Implant instability may also occur when the implant is too small in its overall diameter and is in the vertical position — the 'windshield wiper' syndrome (Fig. 10.5).

The patient complains of changing vision. The implant can be seen moving across the pupil with the position and movement of the head. This problem is likely to arise if the implant is less than 13.5 mm in diameter, where the loops are J-shaped and not a modified J or C shape. A 13.5 or 14 mm implant is unlikely to move in this way particularly if it is positioned horizontally. Any movement is then in a downwards direction. The loops then soon impinge upon the sulcus and achieve stability. The only exception may be in a particularly large eye — such as a myope's. If an implant of the correct design and size is used and it is positioned horizontally then this complication is unlikely. If it does occur then it is possible to fix the lens with a McCannel suture or remove and replace it with a larger size posterior chamber lens.

## Retinal detachment

Retinal detachment is more likely to occur in myopia, where there has been a retinal detachment in the other eye or where there have been vitreous problems such as loss, traction or rupture of the face. The extracapsular approach will reduce the risk of detachment in these patients. Retinal detachment does still occur however and an extracapsular extraction may then create extra difficulties for the retinal surgeon.

An opaque or cloudy capsule, cortical lens remnants, secondary membranes from iritis and residual lens material as well as posterior synechiae and an inadequately dilating pupil may all make it impossible to examine the retina properly. The implant itself may add difficulties either by collecting precipitates on its surfaces or by creating annoying reflections, particularly towards the edge of the optic. Dilation of the pupil may cause a pupillary fixed lens to dislocate and there may be fears that scleral depression will similarly displace a posterior chamber implant.

A perfectly done extracapsular extraction with

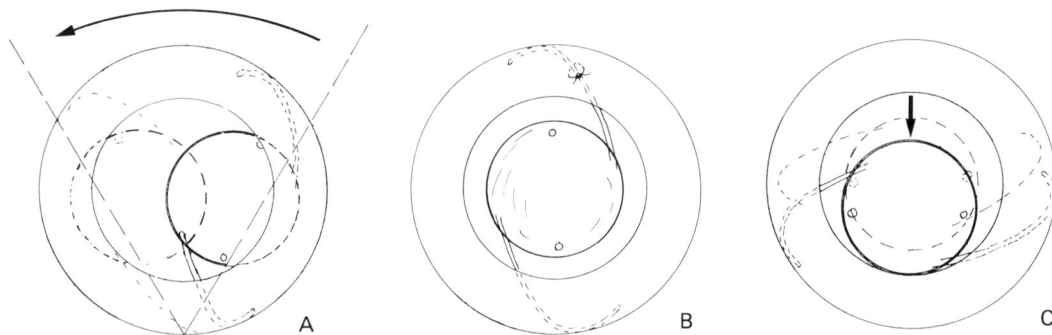

Fig. 10.5 Implant: **A** Unstable in vertical position **B** Loop sutured to iris **C** Stability in horizontal position

or without an implant will be no hindrance to retinal surgery. If all the suggestions presented in this Guide have been followed then the pupil will be free to dilate fully without danger to the stability of the implant; the whole posterior capsule will be transparent because the whole of the anterior capsule has been removed, all the cortical material has been removed and there has been only minimal iritis.

Some posterior capsules will opacify in which case a posterior capsulotomy or capsulectomy must be done. When there has been a rigid pupil then a sector iridectomy will probably have ensured a competent extraction and will allow subsequent fundus examination.

If the extraction has not been adequately performed then further surgery may be necessary to remove membranes or residual lens material. A rigid pupil or one bound down by synechiae will require a sector iridectomy. These procedures may affect the stability of the implant — according to its position and method of fixation. Under these circumstances the implant may have to be removed before adequate retinal surgery can be completed.

Implant surgeons who operate on their own cases of retinal detachment are therefore likely to be less liberal in their indications for implantation than the surgeon who is restricted to the anterior segment. The advantage of the extracapsular method is such that it should be used where detachment of the retina is a risk, and if performed properly is unlikely to cause insurmountable difficulties.

# 11

# Refraction, measurement and astigmatism

The essentials:
- — emmetropia or planned ametropia
- — freedom from astigmatism.

The instruments required:
- — keratometer
- — ultrascan
- — calculator
- — computer.

A technically perfect and uncomplicated procedure has been the goal throughout the previous chapters. There is little point, however, in achieving perfection in technique only to find that the patient — perhaps a first private lens implant or an operation done for a colleague's mother — has 8 dioptres of myopia, 6 dioptres of astigmatism or perhaps 4 dioptres of anisometropia.

Final efforts towards the unattainable must now be directed towards control of the overall refraction by calculation of implant power and control of corneal astigmatism.

## THE REFRACTION

The choice of final refraction for any patient will vary with the individual. Is emmetropia without correction and normal reading glasses preferable to 3 dioptres of planned myopia for easy reading and glasses for distance vision?

It may be more comfortable for a myope to continue with distance glasses, as they have worn them for most of their lives. Someone who is housebound may also find a degree of myopia convenient for vision which is predominantly confined to close range.

The vision and refraction in the nonoperated eye is also important. If the other eye has cataract and poor vision then it may be ignored. If it is free from cataract and has good vision then the implant for the operated eye will have to be calculated to match the refraction of the better eye — otherwise insuperable anisometropia will be the result. Where the nonoperated eye has some degree of cataract then you will have to decide whether to ignore it — assuming that the cataract will soon become complete — or to match it — assuming that there will be useful vision for a worthwhile period of time.

It is no good at all trying to estimate required lens power from the visual acuity, old or new refraction, glasses or history. The more lens implants that you do the more patients you will meet who require implant powers 2, 3 or 4 dioptres different from your estimated normal power. If you do only a few implants you may still be unlucky — or rather your patient will be unlucky, having gone through an operation successfully only to find that vision is poor without correction or that the two eyes cannot be used together.

Soon after I first started doing implants I had a 9 dioptre surprise. The patient had a uniocular cataract. It was not possible to see the fundus and her history appeared to indicate that the eye was normally sighted. The other eye had 6/6 without correction. Facilities for measurement were not then available to me. I implanted a 21 D posterior chamber lens and produced 9 dioptres of myopia.

## MEASUREMENT

Since them I have taken measurements on all patients. It still surprises me to find what odd variations of axial length and corneal curvature combine to produce emmetropia. For example: a woman with a long history of myopia, who had worn glasses since she was 20, had used the same glasses of $-7.75$ D for the last fifteen years. A common rule of thumb which allows 1.5 D of implant power for each 1 D of spectacle error would produce an implant power of 9.5 D for emmetropia.

The measurements were unusual: corneal curvature $K = 41$ D, the axial length $L = 22.75$ mm, and the lens power for emmetropia $P = 23$ D. A 23 D implant was inserted and the final refraction was P1/+1.0 at 180. This was a triumph for measurement over guesswork!

Such unusual measurements are rare. A more frequent finding is that of an unexpectedly long eyeball and flat cornea. A 79-year-old woman is a good example. The eye had a distance correction of $+0.75$ D. The mean corneal curvature $K = 45.5$ D, the axial length $L = 24.3$ mm, and the lens power for emmetropia $P = 15.5$ D. A 15.0 D lens was inserted and the final refraction was $+1.25$ DS. If a standard 21 D implant had been used she would probably have had a final refraction of about $-4.0$ D.

The probability is that without measurement at least 5% of patients will have errors greater than 2 D and 1% will have errors as great as 4 D.

Let us now look at the factors involved in calculating implant power and the effect that errors may have on the final result.

The formula that is easiest to understand is that devised by Sanders, Retzslaf and Kratz — the SRK formula:

$$Pe = A - 2.5L - 0.9K$$

$Pe$ is the predicted lens implant power for emmetropia; $A$ is a constant which has been calculated from a regression formula; $L$ is the axial length of the eyeball measured ultrasonically and expressed in millimetres; and $K$ is the average corneal curvature measured by a keratometer and expressed in dioptres.

This formula is much less complicated than the various theoretical formulae of Binkhorst, Colenbrander and others and is therefore easier to use and check with pencil and paper or a pocket calculator if you do not have easy access to a computer program. The formula was based on the results of several thousand implant operations. The postoperative spectacle errors and depth of anterior chamber were used to calculate what the correct implant power should have been. The constant $A$ was then adjusted according to these results and resubstituted in the formula.

The $A$ constant represents the unknown factor — the postoperative position of the lens implant. This factor will vary with the general type of implant, whether it is designed for the anterior chamber, pre- or postpupillary iris fixation or for the posterior chamber. Posterior chamber lenses of the modified J-loop type, discussed at length in Chapter 8, also show some variation in $A$ constant according to the overall diameter, generally 13, 13.5, 14 and 14.5 mm, and whether the loops are in the same plane as the optic or angled 5, 7 or 10 degrees forward. Construction of the optic also has some effect, whether it is convex anteriorly or so-called reversed optic (convex posterior).

The effect of implant position on the final lens power is relatively small, however. Some $A$ constants published by one manufacturer show a total variation from 117.5 to 115.4 for the complete range of lens types and positions. This difference only produces a variation in implant power of 2.1 D and a variation in spectacle power of about 1.25 D. Nonetheless these are errors to be avoided — and are easily avoided providing that you always use the correct constant for your type of implant. You must be careful when switching from one style to another, for instance for your back-up lens or when trying out new styles. This is another reason why I advise choosing and staying with one lens style and therefore one $A$ constant.

It is then possible to calculate your own individual $A$ constant for further accuracy. The difference may be small but it is worthwhile incorporating in the formula. Thus my own $A$ constant is 117.2 compared with the manufacturer's 116.8. This will produce a difference of about 0.25 D spectacle error. Some published $A$ constants have shown differences of 2.5 between the individual's and the manufacturer's. This would produce a spectacle error of 1.7 D.

The corneal curvature is measured with a keratometer. This is done visually and is a very accurate measurement. The reading can be taken to 0.25 D. An error of 0.25 D will make a difference of only 0.22 D in implant power and a spectacle error of 0.13 D. Errors in $K$ readings will thus have only a small effect on the total calculation. Errors in keratometry do occur, however, from difficulties in fixation by the patient. The measurement should be taken along the visual axis and thus refer only to 2 or 3 mm of the central cornea. If the patient is unable to see the fixation light, as in the presence of a mature cataract, or is unable to take up or maintain fixation owing to physical or mental infirmity, then your measurement may not be taken from the correct part of the cornea. If accuracy is essential, it is possible to take the measurement under anaesthetic, but alignment with the true visual axis may still be at fault.

Irregular astigmatism from scarring or degeneration may make keratometry most unreliable, but is fortunately not too common. Regular astigmatism is common however. The SRK formula requires a single figure for the $K$ reading. An average figure is therefore taken between the readings from the two axes of astigmatism. If the degree of astigmatism is large or if it changes with the healing of the wound then the final refraction may be difficult to predict and may be some way from that desired.

Measurement of the axial length is made using an ultrasonic scanner. An error of 1 mm will alter the predicted implant power by 2.5 D and produce a spectacle error of 1.6 D. This is a large error and the ultrasonic scan thus becomes the most important error factor in the formula. The measurement is made by bringing the diagnostic probe into contact with the cornea in a fluid medium. The instrument is aligned along the visual axis and a reading taken from the cornea to the retinal surface. Early instruments achieved contact through an open water bath but later instruments are much easier to manipulate with the use of a thin membrane, which separates the fluid from the cornea, or an all-solid probe. The instruments require careful preparation, setting up and calibration. There is then the difficulty of aligning the visual axis, especially in the poorly seeing eye. Reliable measurements can only be achieved through regular use and practice.

The calculation is easy. The measured values and $A$ constant are substituted in the formula and $Pe$ obtained. Simple errors of transposition and arithmetic are possible and do occasionally occur. My Registrar and I work out the implant powers separately and then compare them. These types of error can be reduced if a calculator is used and can be reduced almost to zero with a preprogrammed computer.

Fortunately there are now several instruments available which are much easier to use. They incorporate a multiple measuring and recording device so that a series of measurements is taken. The machine is able to discard inaccurate measurements and present a mean of those taken. One can thus be certain that probe pressure was not too great, that the system was bubble free and alignment along the visual axis was correct. Such machines are or can be programmed to accept other data for various lens power calculations, for instance for a back-up lens. The whole measurement and calculation will only take a few minutes and can be relied upon for accuracy and freedom from error. They are of course expensive.

The standard SRK formula is used in a modified form when a degree of ametropia is required. It now becomes:

$$Pa = A - 2.5L - 0.9K - 1.25R$$

$R$ is the desired spectacle correction and $Pa$ the predicted implant power that will produce this error.

An example is provided by a 45-year-old woman who had a mature cataract in one eye which developed several years after a shuttlecock injury. Her good eye had 6/5 vision with $-3.25/+1.25$ at 90 (spherical equivalent $-2.63$ D). The measurements for the cataractous eye were $K = 42.75$ and $L = 24.52$. The calculation using an $A$ constant of 116.8 gave an implant power of 17.0 D for emmetropia and 21.25 ametropia of $-2.75$ D.

$$Pe = 116.8 - 2.5(24.52) - 0.9(42.75)$$
$$= 17.00$$
$$Pa = 116.8 - 2.5(24.52) - 0.9(42.75) - 1.25(-2.63) = 21.00$$

A 21.0 D implant was used and her final refraction was $-4.0/+1.25$ at 180, a spherical equivalent of about $-3.38$ D.

Calculation of one's own $A$ constant is a worth-while task. By making use of data from patients measured and operated on in one's own department, any differences in the standardization or calibration of the instruments in addition to individual differences in the use of the instruments and in one's own particular surgical technique can be compensated for in the $A$ constant, thus leading to greater accuracy. The procedure for the calculation is as follows.

Record the $K$ readings, the axial length, post-operative refraction (spherical equivalent) and actual power of implant used. Calculate the predicted power that would give the postoperative spherical equivalent. Take the difference between this and the actual power implanted. Add this difference to the $A$ constant used. This figure is the new $A$ constant for this particular patient.

An example will make this clearer:

$K = 46.75$
$L = 24.0$
Postoperative refraction $= +0.75$ D
Implant used $= 15.0$ D

Predicted implant power for spectacle error of $+0.75$ is 14.2 D ($Pi = A - 2.5L - 0.9K - 1.25R$). Difference between actual implant power and predicted implant power is $+0.8$. The revised $A$ constant is therefore:

$116.8 + 0.8 = 117.8.$

In practice, the more data that can be incorporated, the more accurate will be the $A$ constant. It is sensible however to discard any results which show large deviations as these are probably caused by large errors in measurement.

Calculation and use of one's own $A$ constant is a good way of keeping in touch with postoperative results and as at least 100 patients are needed it maintains some degree of conservatism in the approach to implant choice.

## ASTIGMATISM

Discussion of astigmatism can be confusing. Corneal astigmatism may be qualified by reference to its meridian of greater or lesser curvature or by reference to its axis. Sometimes, however,

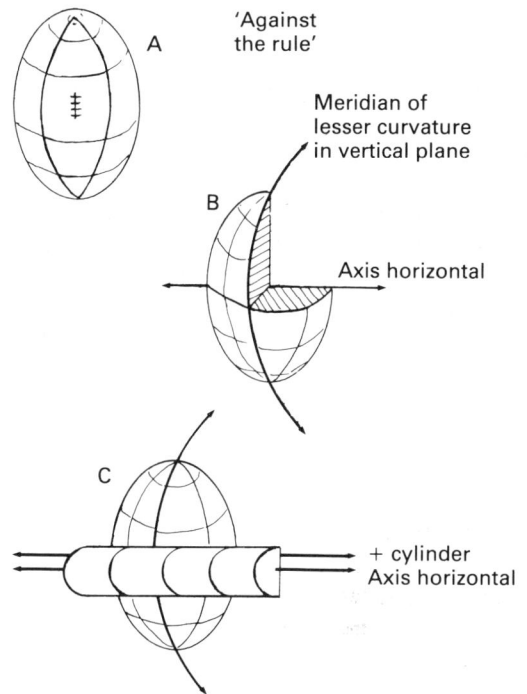

Fig. 11.1 Astigmatism: **A** Rugby ball on its tip **B** Meridian of lesser curvature is in the vertical plane. Axis of lesser curvature is horizontal **C** Correction of lesser curvature by + cylinder axis horizontal. Astigmatism 'against the rule'

discussion about the correction of astigmatism refers to the cylindrical lens which is used and the direction of its axis. Greater confusion arises because plus or minus cylinders may be used for this correction (Fig. 11.1).

The astigmatic cornea can readily be compared with a rugby ball. I find this image helpful when trying to see how astigmatism is produced and how it may be corrected.

Let us first imagine that the rugby ball is standing on its end. The flatter meridian, of lesser curvature, is the vertical one. The axis of this meridian is horizontal. It would be corrected by a plus cylinder with its axis horizontal — at 180 degrees in the trial frame. This type of astigmatism is often called 'against the rule'.

'With the rule' means that the cornea is flattened in the horizontal meridian. It is corrected optically by a plus cylinder with its axis at 90 degrees. The rugby ball is horizontal.

The degree of astigmatism is less than 1.25 D in over 80% of people. Errors of greater than

2.5 D against the rule or 6.0 D with the rule are relatively rare in otherwise normal eyes.

The axis and to some extent the degree of astigmatism change with age so that by the age of 80 years 85% have astigmatism against the rule.

The corneoscleral incision for cataract surgery has a profound effect upon corneal astigmatism. The main purposes of the incision must be recalled before various aspects of this are considered. It must allow adequate access for the planned surgical manoeuvres. At the same time it must be watertight when closed. There must also be minimal interference with the normal functions of the eye. If these important criteria are not remembered and put into practice effectively then complications far more important than some few dioptres of residual astigmatism are likely to occur.

The healing of what we may call an average cataract incision will be known to most surgeons who have followed the refraction of their patients in the first few postoperative weeks (Fig. 11.2). My own average incision for an intracapsular extraction is large, 170 degrees. It is sutured by five to seven, 8–0 virgin silk interrupted sutures. The refraction is very variable during the first four to five days. By the sixth day there is usually 2–4 D of astigmatism 'with the rule'. During the

next three weeks the axis of astigmatism swings through 90 degrees and the power becomes less. At eight weeks the final figure is attained. The astigmatism is between 0 and 2 D 'against the rule' and is therefore corrected by a plus cylinder at 180 degrees. The range is much greater and rarely may exceed 6 D. This range of results depends partly on the degree and direction of preoperative astigmatism.

When the incision is smaller, 90–120 degrees, as used for an extracapsular cataract extraction, the astigmatism behaves in much the same way, but the changes are smaller.

When the incision is small, 3–4 mm, as used in phakoemulsification, the changes are different. The astigmatism is less from the time of the operation. It is initially with the rule. It becomes less but may never go against the rule.

There are a number of general factors that should be discussed before the ways in which astigmatism can be modified are to be considered.

The position of the incision is important. A corneal incision induces more astigmatism. It is also slower to heal, but is very comfortable for the patient.

The scleral incision heals with less astigmatism and more quickly. It bleeds more readily and is more painful for the patient. An incision far back

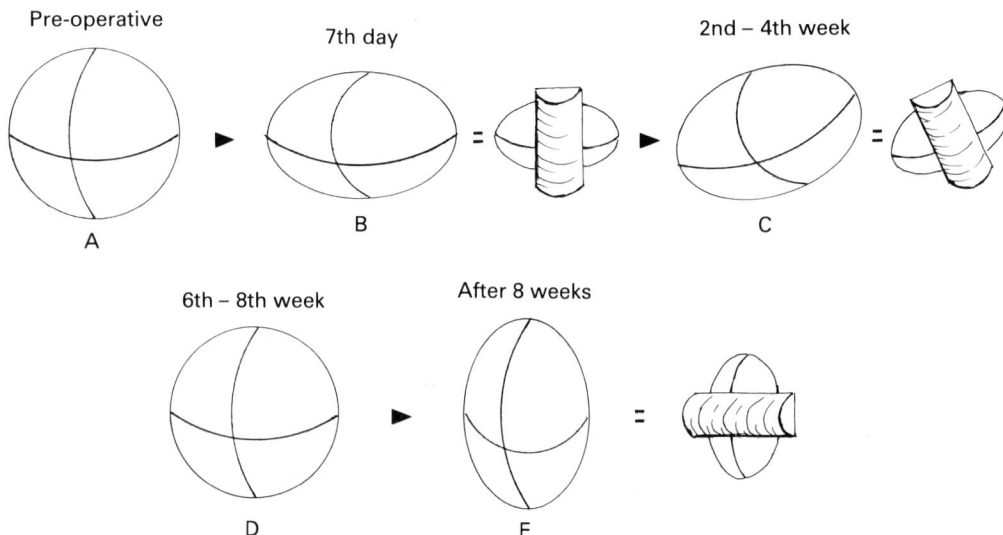

**Fig. 11.2** Astigmatism — post operative changes: **A** Spherical before operation **B** Seventh day — curvature of vertical meridian increased **C** Second to fourth week — axis changes towards horizontal **D** Sixth to eighth week — return to spherical state **E** After eighth week — vertical meridian becomes flatter

on the sclera has to be modified in order to open into the eye without interfering with the drainage angle and iris root.

The construction of the incision is important both for astigmatism and adequate wound closure. A forward shelving incision is unstable and allows the two sides of the wound to slide apart or to overlap. Back shelving incisions or incisions constructed in two or three planes overcome this problem. They are stable, watertight and reduce astigmatism.

The method of closure also has an important effect. Single interrupted sutures are perhaps the safest to maintain a watertight wound but offer more chance of a stitch being too tight or too loose. A continuous suture will distribute tension equally along the length of the incision but may be slightly more difficult to tie with the correct tension.

The suture material is significant. Nonabsorbable material allows complete healing of the incision while constant suture tension is maintained — providing they are tied sufficiently tight, do not come untied or cut out. Absorbable materials, even those with the longest lives, will have lost most if not all of their tensile strength by the end of the sixth week. This is long before the incision has healed and before astigmatism has become stable.

All of these general factors may have a considerable effect on the result in any individual patient. It is necessary to develop your own 'standard' incision with regard to these factors before you can contemplate controlling or modifying astigmatism. So stick to the same combination of position, construction, closure and suture material until your results are consistent.

Two examples serve to illustrate some of the problems that our patients may have.

A 45-year-old woman had developed a mature cataract in one eye 15 years after a shuttlecock injury. She had a cataract extraction and implant calculated to match her normal eye. Three months later her refraction was:

| | | |
|---|---|---|
| Normal eye | $-3.25/+1.25$ at 90 | 6/5 |
| Operated eye | $-4.0/+1.25$ at 180 | 6/5 |

The preoperative $K$ readings were $K1$ 42 at 0 and $K2$ 43.50 at 90.

This change of 2.5 D in power and 90 degree in angle caused her to complain of tilting of horizontal lines and some feeling of disorientation. Fortunately these symptoms became gradually less troublesome.

The second example was a 49-year-old man who had a penetrating corneoscleral injury and traumatic cataract. A difficult extraction and implant successfully restored 6/9 vision. This enabled him

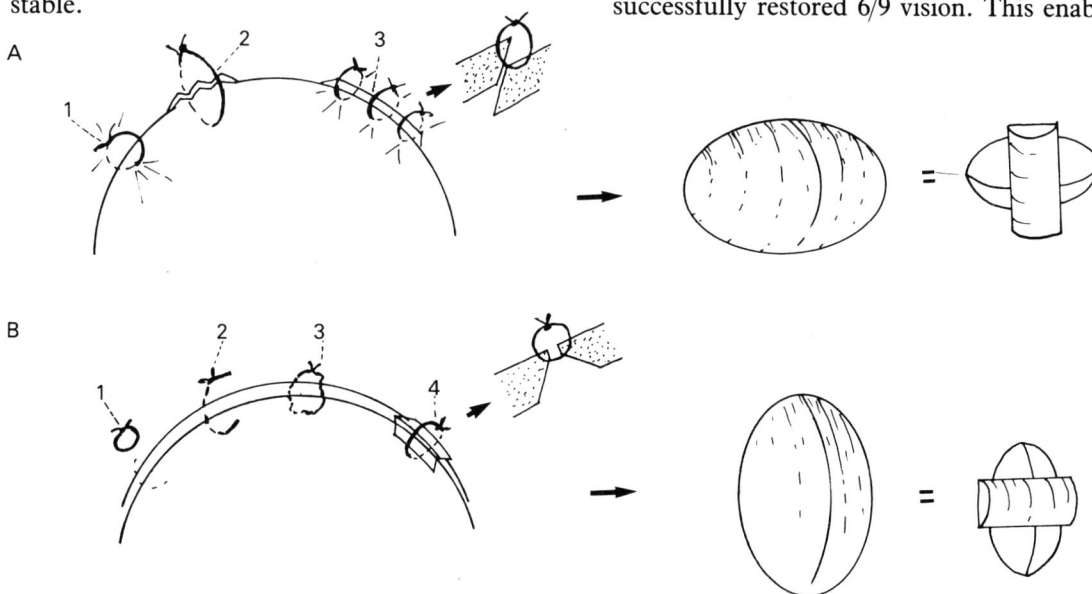

**Fig. 11.3** Astigmatism: **A** Steepening of vertical meridian 1. Suture too tight 2. Suture bite too long 3. Wound edges overriding **B** Flattening of vertical meridian 1. Suture cuts out 2. Suture broken 3. Suture too loose 4. Suture too superficial

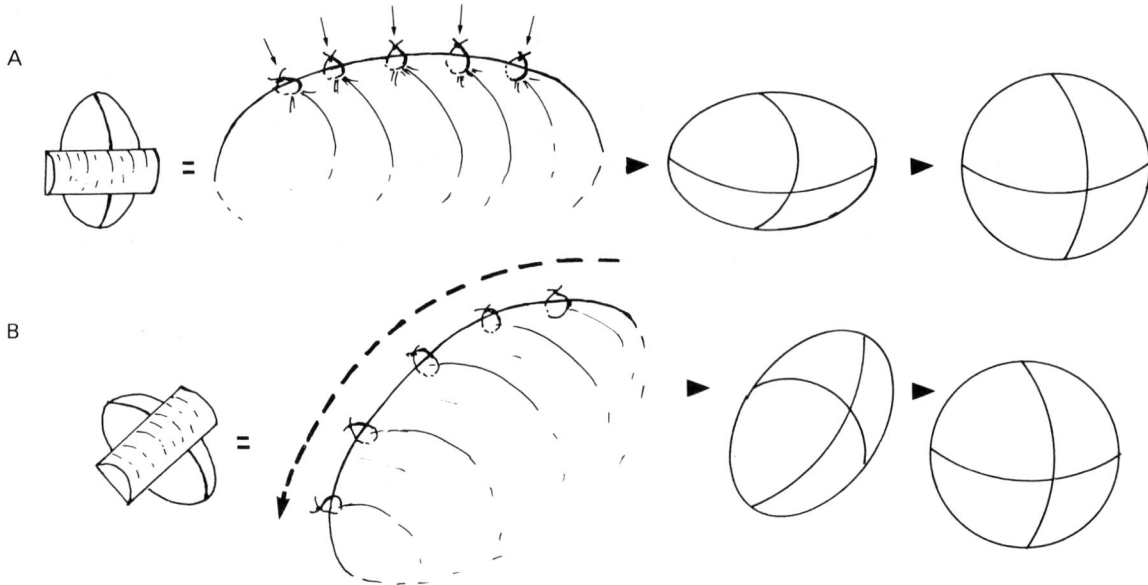

**Fig. 11.4** Astigmatism — control: **A** Correct 'against the rule' astigmatism by steepening steep vertical meridian with tight sutures **B** Correct oblique astigmatism by position of incision

to retain his job. Unfortunately he was left with 4.5 D of astigmatism and could not wear the spectacle correction comfortably. In this instance the astigmatism was caused by the corneal injury and was not fully corrected by the cataract incision.

Such problems may not seem too important for most cataract patients, especially when cataract is present in both eyes. As one's indications for lens implantation become wider, however, the need for control of astigmatism becomes more necessary and the near perfect result not quite good enough.

Attempts to correct astigmatism may be made at the time of the operation, within the first few postoperative weeks — during which the incision is still healing — or some time after the incision has fully healed.

At the time of the operation an incision between nine and three o'clock may cause the cornea to steepen in the vertical meridian — the rugby football in the horizontal position — if the stitches are tied too tightly, if the suture bites are too broad allowing the wound edge to buckle or if the wound edges are allowed to ride over one another (Fig. 11.3).

The cornea may flatten in the vertical meridian — the rugby ball now in the vertical position — if the stitches are tied too loosely, if a stitch comes untied or cuts through or if the stitch is

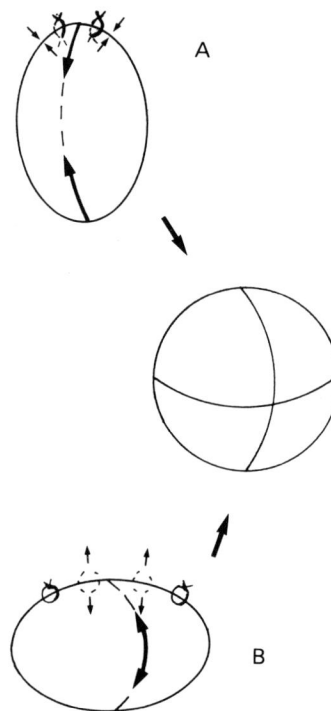

**Fig. 11.5** Astigmatism — control: **A** Steepen vertical meridian by tightening sutures **B** Flatten vertical meridian by cutting sutures

placed too superficially, allowing the internal part of the incision to gape.

Stitches that are too loose or too superficial are to be avoided as they may affect proper wound healing. Alteration of astigmatism may therefore be effected by suitably tightening one or more sutures at selected sites along the length of the incision. Further control can be achieved by positioning the incision more nasally or more temporally to suit a particular axis of astigmatism (Fig. 11.4). In general one should not tie the sutures too tightly. A method is needed to monitor the overall effect of suture tightness on the incision. Such methods range from use of a simple air bubble, corneal reflections or the complicated and expensive operation keratometer.

Between the fourth and sixth postoperative weeks astigmatism may be altered by the cutting or removal of one or more sutures (Fig. 11.5).

Once the incision has completely healed change can only be brought about by selectively resecting an appropriate wedge of cornea.

It is only fair to say that my efforts to control astigmatism have had variable and not always satisfying results.

# Index